Creatine Uncovered:
The Hidden Power
Behind Health, Brain, and Longevity

Creatine Uncovered: The Hidden Power Behind Health, Brain, and Longevity

Rex Nihilo

Creatine Uncovered: The Hidden Power Behind Health, Brain, and Longevity
Copyright © 2025 by Rex Nihilo

First Edition: 2025

ISBN: 978-1-997668-50-3

Cover design by The Author
Printed in USA

Disclaimer: The information in this book is provided for general educational purposes only. Please see full disclaimer.

Creatine Uncovered: The Hidden Power Behind Health, Brain, and Longevity

Rex Nihilo

"The currency of life is energy. The more you have, the more you can do, be, and experience."

— *Dr. Mark Hyman*, physician and functional medicine expert

"We are not programmed to decline. We are programmed to repair. Aging is optional."

— *Dr. David Sinclair*, Harvard longevity researcher and author of *Lifespan: Why We Age—and Why We Don't Have To*

"Muscle is the organ of longevity."

— *Dr. Gabrielle Lyon*, physician and expert in muscle-centric medicine

---

"Creatine is one of the most well-researched supplements in existence, with benefits extending far beyond athletic performance."

— *Dr. Jose Antonio*, PhD, CEO of the International Society of Sports Nutrition

Disclaimer

The information presented in this book, *"Creatine Uncovered: The Hidden Power Behind Health, Brain, and Longevity,"* is intended for educational and informational purposes only. It is not intended to serve as a substitute for professional medical advice, diagnosis, or treatment.

While every effort has been made to ensure the accuracy and validity of the content, readers are strongly advised to consult with a licensed physician, registered dietitian, or qualified healthcare provider before beginning any new supplement regimen, especially if they have pre-existing medical conditions, are pregnant or breastfeeding, are taking medications, or are undergoing medical treatment.

The authors and contributors of this book are not liable for any damages or adverse effects arising from the use or misuse of the information provided herein.

Creatine supplementation, while supported by a large body of scientific research, may not be suitable for everyone. Always follow recommended dosing and safety guidelines as outlined by reputable health organizations.

Acknowledgment of AI Assistance

This book was developed with the assistance of advanced artificial intelligence tools, including OpenAI's GPT-4o model. AI was utilized throughout the research, drafting, organization, editing, and fact-checking processes to enhance clarity, structure, and accessibility for general readers.

Final content decisions, interpretations of research, and overall editorial oversight were made by the human author or user commissioning this work. AI tools were used as support, not as a replacement for scientific review or personal judgment.

This acknowledgment is provided in the spirit of transparency, integrity, and responsible use of emerging technologies in publishing.

Introduction: Creatine – The Quiet Revolution in Modern Health

In the world of health and wellness, certain nutrients have always taken center stage - vitamins like C and D, minerals like calcium and iron, and macronutrients like protein and fiber. Yet quietly, and often misunderstood, one compound has been steadily building its case for becoming the most important health supplement of the 21st century: **creatine monohydrate**.

For decades, creatine has been pigeonholed as a muscle-building supplement, the staple of weightlifters and athletes. It was celebrated in locker rooms and fitness magazines yet largely ignored by the broader medical community and public. But that narrative is now shifting - rapidly and radically.

Recent breakthroughs in human physiology, neuroscience, and clinical nutrition have revealed a vastly more complex and exciting picture. Far from being just "a gym supplement," creatine is now emerging as a **powerful, multi-system support molecule** - capable of influencing everything from brain function and mental health to bone density, cardiovascular performance, aging, and even pregnancy outcomes.

What makes creatine unique is not just the **breadth of its benefits**, but the **depth of scientific validation** supporting it. Between 2020 and 2025, a surge of research has confirmed that creatine supplementation can:

- Boost memory and attention span
- Improve mood and reduce depression symptoms
- Protect against neurodegeneration
- Enhance heart function and lower triglycerides
- Reduce the loss of bone density with age
- Help maintain muscle mass and function in older adults
- Improve recovery from injuries and mental fatigue
- Safely support health during menstruation, pregnancy, and menopause

What's even more compelling is that creatine is **naturally present in the human body**, produced in the liver, kidneys, and pancreas, and obtained from foods like red meat and fish. However, many people - especially women, older adults, vegetarians, and those under metabolic stress - do not get enough. For them, supplementation offers **profound health improvements**, both immediate and long-term.

And despite persistent myths, creatine has one of the **most robust safety profiles** in the supplement world. Numerous studies confirm that even high doses taken over long periods **do not harm kidney or liver function** in healthy individuals. Side effects, when they occur, are rare and mild.

This book is written not for bodybuilders or elite athletes - but for **you**. Whether you're a student looking to enhance mental clarity, a parent seeking better energy and mood, an older adult aiming to stay mobile, or someone simply wanting to thrive through all stages of life - **this guide will walk you through the transformative potential of creatine**.

We will dive into the science, yes - but with simplicity and clarity. Each chapter is designed to uncover one of creatine's powerful benefits, guided by real studies, practical advice, and personalized insights for different lifestyles and age groups.

In the pages ahead, you'll learn:

- How creatine works at the cellular level to regenerate energy
- Why its effects on the brain may rival those of nootropics
- How it helps women during the hormonal rollercoaster of life
- Why doctors are now looking at creatine for managing diabetes, arthritis, and even depression

By the end of this book, you'll see creatine not just as a supplement - but as a **cornerstone of modern health strategy**. One that belongs in conversations about longevity, vitality, and prevention - not just performance.

Welcome to the quiet revolution of creatine. It's time to uncover the science, embrace the benefits, and reimagine your health with one of nature's most powerful allies.

Chapter 1: The Forgotten Molecule - Why Creatine Deserves a Second Look

For most people, the word *creatine* instantly evokes images of gym-goers gulping down shakes, aspiring bodybuilders piling on muscle mass, and athletes aiming for that competitive edge. It's long been associated almost exclusively with sports performance. And while it's true that creatine plays a powerful role in physical strength and muscle endurance, this narrow perception has done the molecule a great disservice.

Because behind the protein-shake stereotypes lies one of the most fascinating, well-researched, and *misunderstood* compounds in human health. Creatine is no longer just a performance enhancer; it's a foundational cellular compound that touches nearly every system in the human body. In this chapter, we'll explore why creatine deserves a second look - and why this naturally occurring molecule may be the most important supplement you've never truly considered.

A Brief History of Creatine's Reputation

Creatine was first identified in the early 1800s by French scientist Michel Eugène Chevreul. Its name comes from the Greek word *kreas*, meaning meat, due to its concentration in muscle-rich foods like beef and fish. But it wasn't until the 1990s that creatine burst into mainstream consciousness as a legal and effective way to enhance athletic performance. Athletes at the 1992 Barcelona Olympics credited creatine supplementation for their strength gains, and by the late 90s, it was widely available over the counter.

From then on, creatine was stuck with an identity: a *muscle supplement*. The sports world loved it. The medical community? Less so. Skepticism was rampant. Was it safe? Was it just a fad? Did it damage kidneys? Much of the early discourse was shaped by anecdote, misinformation, and a lack of high-quality clinical data.

But that has changed. Fast forward to today, and the story of creatine is being rewritten.

A Cellular Powerhouse

To understand why creatine matters, you need to look beyond muscle mass and athletic prowess and dive into the heart of cellular biology. At its core, creatine is about *energy* - not just physical energy, but cellular energy that fuels every organ, every tissue, every moment of your life.

The body stores creatine in two forms: free creatine and phosphocreatine. The latter plays a critical role in regenerating adenosine triphosphate (ATP), the body's primary energy currency. During periods of intense activity - whether you're lifting a dumbbell, sprinting across a street, or solving a complex problem - ATP is rapidly depleted. Phosphocreatine helps recycle it almost instantaneously.

This energy buffering system is especially vital in "energy-hungry" tissues like muscles and the brain. That's why creatine is stored not just in skeletal muscle, but in the brain, where it supports mental endurance, memory, and neurological resilience. And that's just the beginning.

From Muscle Supplement to Multi-System Optimizer

Modern research has unveiled creatine's impact across multiple domains of health:

- **Brain Health**: Studies show creatine can enhance memory, reduce mental fatigue, and even protect against neurodegeneration.
- **Mental Health**: Creatine may help alleviate depression and support recovery from traumatic brain injuries.
- **Bone Health**: Creatine boosts osteoblast activity and may reduce bone resorption, aiding in the prevention of fractures.

- **Cardiovascular Health**: It improves vascular function, reduces triglycerides, and supports endothelial health.
- **Metabolic Support**: Creatine may aid in glucose regulation and reduce markers of metabolic disease.
- **Healthy Aging**: For older adults, creatine can slow or reverse sarcopenia, support cognitive function, and enhance balance and mobility.

This evolution in understanding has led scientists and physicians to rethink creatine entirely. No longer just an ergogenic aid for athletes, it's now being positioned as a *nutraceutical* - a dietary compound with potential clinical applications.

Creatine Deficiency in the General Population

Surprisingly, many people - especially those who don't consume animal products - are creatine-deficient. Our bodies do produce creatine naturally (about 1-2 grams per day), but dietary intake is also crucial. Red meat, fish, and poultry are primary sources. As a result, **vegans and vegetarians often have lower muscle and brain creatine levels**, leading to more pronounced benefits from supplementation.

Additionally, women tend to have lower baseline creatine stores than men, and this discrepancy grows during pregnancy, menopause, and other life stages. Older adults, too, experience declining creatine levels due to reduced muscle mass and dietary shifts.

In other words, the people who may *need* creatine the most - women, older adults, vegans - are often the least likely to get enough from their diets.

Debunking the Myths

For all of its benefits, creatine has been the target of persistent myths. Perhaps the most common? That it damages your kidneys.

The confusion stems from the fact that creatine supplementation raises levels of creatinine, a byproduct that is *also* a biomarker for kidney function. But elevated creatinine from supplementation doesn't indicate kidney damage - it simply reflects increased creatine metabolism. **In healthy individuals, creatine has shown no adverse effects on kidney or liver function**, even at high doses over extended periods.

Another myth is that creatine causes water retention or bloating. While creatine does increase intracellular water (hydrating your muscles from within), it doesn't typically cause visible or uncomfortable bloating. In fact, this hydration may be beneficial, especially for older adults.

Why the Medical Community is Finally Taking Notice

In the last five years, research into creatine has exploded. From neurology journals to clinical nutrition conferences, creatine is finally being taken seriously by scientists and doctors alike.

Why now?

1. **Wider Health Context**: As chronic diseases become more prevalent, healthcare is shifting focus from treatment to prevention. Creatine fits perfectly into this model.
2. **Robust Research**: Dozens of randomized controlled trials now support its benefits across various conditions.
3. **Aging Population**: As the global population ages, creatine offers a safe, affordable tool to combat sarcopenia, dementia, and falls.

4. **Mental Health Crisis**: With growing rates of depression and cognitive decline, creatine's neuroprotective and mood-stabilizing effects are more relevant than ever.

Leading researchers are calling for creatine to be considered in clinical settings - not just supplement stores. It's a shift from niche to mainstream.

Why You Should Care

Whether you're 25 or 75, an athlete or office worker, omnivore or vegan - creatine may offer benefits that matter to your everyday life:

- Want more energy during your day? Creatine helps.
- Battling brain fog or poor memory? Creatine helps.
- Trying to stay strong, fit, and independent as you age? Creatine helps.
- Recovering from illness, injury, or emotional burnout? Creatine helps.

The most compelling part? **It's affordable, accessible, and backed by science**.

The New Paradigm

What's emerging is a new paradigm: creatine as a **broad-spectrum health optimizer**, not just a sports supplement. It supports energy production, cellular repair, gene regulation, antioxidant defense, and more. And because of its safety and versatility, it's quickly becoming one of the most promising tools in the modern health arsenal.

We are standing at the edge of a quiet revolution in preventative and integrative medicine - and creatine is at the center of it.

Coming Up Next

In Chapter 2, we'll explore how creatine fuels the body - diving deep into how the **creatine-phosphocreatine system** works and why this ATP-regenerating mechanism is essential for *every aspect* of movement, muscle, and even recovery.

Chapter 2: Fueling the Body - How Creatine Powers Muscles and Movement

If you've ever sprinted up a flight of stairs, pushed through a tough workout, or even carried groceries to your car, you've relied on one of the body's most powerful but often overlooked energy systems: the **creatine-phosphocreatine system**. This biological pathway is responsible for generating quick, explosive energy - when you need it most.

While muscles often steal the spotlight in creatine discussions, what really deserves our attention is *how* creatine enables movement, performance, and endurance at a cellular level. In this chapter, we explore the fascinating mechanism behind creatine's energy support role, and how it translates into real-world gains - whether you're an athlete or just trying to age well.

The Body's Energy Currency: ATP

To appreciate creatine's function, we first need to understand **adenosine triphosphate (ATP)**, often called the body's energy currency.

ATP is the molecule that powers nearly every physiological function - muscle contraction, nerve impulse transmission, nutrient transport, even thinking. When you move your arm or blink your eye, your cells are using ATP.

But there's a catch: **cells can store only a small amount of ATP**, and during intense activity, this supply is depleted in seconds. Your body must continuously regenerate ATP to maintain function. And this is where creatine steps in.

Meet the Creatine-Phosphocreatine System

Creatine exists in two main forms inside the cell:

1. **Free creatine**
2. **Phosphocreatine (PCr)** – the high-energy form, created when a phosphate group attaches to creatine

The creatine-phosphocreatine system works as a rapid energy buffer. When your body uses ATP and breaks it down into **adenosine diphosphate (ADP)**, phosphocreatine steps up, donating its phosphate to regenerate ATP - quickly and efficiently.

This regeneration process is especially critical during:

- Sprinting
- Weightlifting
- Jumping
- Any short burst of high-intensity activity

This system can sustain maximum energy output for about **6 to 10 seconds** - the difference between completing a final push or collapsing in exhaustion.

Why This Matters for Physical Performance

Let's say you're doing resistance training and you hit 8 reps on a bench press. With more creatine stored in your muscles, you might push through to 10 reps. Those two extra reps may not sound like much, but over weeks and months, this adds up to greater muscle growth, strength, and endurance.

Clinical studies have shown that creatine supplementation:

- Increases **lean body mass** by an average of **1.32 kg**
- Boosts **upper-body strength** by over **4 kg**
- Improves **lower-body strength** by over **11 kg**
- Enhances **anaerobic capacity** (e.g., sprint performance, jumping)
- Speeds up **muscle recovery** between intense bouts of exercise

But beyond just "lifting more," creatine allows for **higher training volume** - more sets, more reps, less fatigue - which accelerates adaptations like hypertrophy and strength gains.

The "Spatial Energy Buffer": Creatine's Mitochondrial Connection

The creatine system isn't just a short-term fix. It also connects two major cellular power systems: mitochondrial respiration (long-term energy production) and cytosolic energy needs (sudden bursts). Scientists call this a **spatial energy buffer**.

Here's what happens:

- Mitochondria produce ATP during aerobic metabolism.
- Creatine accepts a phosphate group in the mitochondria, becoming phosphocreatine.
- Phosphocreatine diffuses through the cell, storing that energy.
- When needed, it donates the phosphate to ADP, regenerating ATP where it's urgently required - like at the site of muscle contraction.

This buffering keeps ATP levels high and ADP levels low, maintaining **cellular energy homeostasis**. That's a fancy way of saying your cells stay "fueled and ready."

Creatine's Role in Recovery and Reduced Fatigue

One of the most underappreciated benefits of creatine is its impact on **exercise recovery**. It's not just about helping you perform - it's about helping you perform again, and again, with less breakdown.

Here's how:

- **Delays fatigue**: By buffering hydrogen ions (H^+), creatine reduces muscle acidosis, which is partly responsible for the burning sensation and fatigue during exercise.
- **Reduces muscle damage**: Supplementation has been shown to lower levels of **creatine kinase**, a marker of muscle damage.
- **Shortens relaxation time**: Muscles relax and recover more quickly after contraction.
- **Improves satellite cell activity**: These are essential for muscle repair and growth.
- **Supports anti-catabolic action**: Creatine may help reduce muscle protein breakdown after exercise.

All of these effects contribute to faster and more complete recovery, allowing you to **train more frequently and effectively**.

Resistance Training + Creatine = Synergy

Creatine's benefits are significantly amplified when combined with **resistance training**. This combo creates a perfect storm for muscle adaptation. In fact, it's one of the **few supplements consistently shown to enhance the effects of strength training** across age groups.

In older adults, for example, the synergy is remarkable:

- Creatine supplementation + resistance training = **improved mobility**, **greater strength**, **increased lean mass**, and **reduced risk of falls**.
- This dual approach has been shown to **reverse sarcopenia**, the age-related loss of muscle and strength.

In younger populations, it enables:

- Faster progression in training programs
- Higher energy output in sports and physical performance
- Enhanced body composition

In both cases, **creatine doesn't replace exercise - it supercharges it.**

Creatine for Everyday Movement and Physical Function

Even if you never set foot in a gym, creatine still plays a vital role in your daily movement and stamina. Think of these common scenarios:

- Climbing stairs without losing breath
- Carrying groceries or a toddler
- Standing up from a seated position
- Walking longer distances without fatigue

These basic movements rely on quick bursts of energy and neuromuscular coordination - all of which benefit from optimal creatine stores.

This is especially relevant for **older adults**, who often experience declines in:

- Muscle mass and power
- Balance and coordination

- Recovery from minor injuries or fatigue

Creatine supplementation in this population has shown **consistent improvements in mobility, strength, and balance**, contributing to greater independence and quality of life.

What About Endurance?

Creatine is most famous for short, high-intensity efforts - but emerging research shows potential benefits in **endurance sports** too:

- Enhances **interval training** by speeding recovery between bursts
- May increase **glycogen storage** in muscles
- Potentially reduces inflammation and oxidative stress after prolonged exertion

Though it's not a replacement for endurance-focused nutrition like carbohydrates and electrolytes, creatine can serve as a **supporting supplement** - especially for athletes engaging in high-volume, mixed-modality training like CrossFit, cycling, or team sports.

Muscle Creatine Saturation: Why It Matters

You might be wondering: how does creatine actually accumulate in the muscle?

Muscle tissue is like a sponge - it absorbs and stores creatine, but only to a limit. This is called **muscle creatine saturation**. Once the sponge is full, any extra creatine is simply excreted. That's why **regular, consistent supplementation** is important.

There are two common strategies:

1. **Loading Phase**: 20 grams/day (split into 4 doses) for 5-7 days to quickly saturate muscle
2. **Gradual Approach**: 3-5 grams/day for 3-4 weeks to slowly achieve the same saturation

Once saturation is reached, a **maintenance dose of 3-5 grams per day** is enough to keep levels optimal.

You don't have to cycle on and off. Creatine is **safe for long-term use**, and studies show its effects persist as long as saturation is maintained.

Summary: Why Creatine Powers More Than Performance

Creatine is not just about building biceps or sprinting faster - it's a **cornerstone of muscular energy**, cellular health, and physical resilience. Its ability to regenerate ATP, buffer fatigue, enhance recovery, and support daily function makes it indispensable for:

- Athletes of all levels
- Older adults aiming to stay strong
- Busy professionals looking to reduce fatigue
- Anyone trying to move better, live longer, and feel more energized

Whether you're lifting weights, hiking a trail, or just trying to keep up with life, **creatine powers the engine that keeps you going**.

Coming Up Next

In Chapter 3: Beyond Energy — The Cellular Magic of Creatine, we'll uncover how creatine influences gene expression, antioxidant defense, inflammation, and mitochondrial health—unlocking its role as a full-spectrum cellular protector, not just an energy booster.

Chapter 3: Beyond Energy - The Cellular Magic of Creatine

Unlocking its hidden roles in genetic expression, antioxidant defense, and inflammation control

For most of its modern history, creatine has been described as a molecule with one purpose: energy. And while it's true that creatine's ability to regenerate ATP is at the heart of its ergogenic effects, we now know that this compound is far more than an energy booster. In fact, its presence in various tissues - especially the brain, bones, and even immune cells - points to a **multifunctional role in maintaining cellular health and resilience**.

This chapter uncovers the emerging science of how creatine acts as a **cellular guardian**, influencing gene regulation, protecting cells from oxidative stress, and even fine-tuning inflammation. These "non-energy" benefits are not just side effects - they may very well be the foundation of creatine's broad health impact.

1. Creatine as a Molecular Signal: Influencing Gene Expression

Perhaps one of the most remarkable findings in recent creatine research is its ability to **modulate gene expression**.

Genes are like switches, turned on or off depending on signals within the cell. These signals come from hormones, nutrients, and even stressors. Creatine, it turns out, can act as one of these **molecular messengers**. By influencing genetic activity, it affects the creation of proteins that regulate growth, repair, and inflammation.

Studies have shown that creatine may upregulate genes associated with:

- **Muscle growth** (via IGF-1 and myogenic regulatory factors)
- **Cell survival** under metabolic stress
- **Mitochondrial biogenesis**, or the formation of new energy-producing mitochondria
- **Antioxidant defenses**, such as glutathione-related enzymes

This means creatine doesn't just help you perform better today - it may help **reprogram your cells for resilience** over the long term.

---

2. Mitochondrial Support: The Cell's Power Grid

Mitochondria are the **energy plants** of your cells, converting nutrients into ATP through aerobic respiration. They are also critical for:

- Cell signaling
- Calcium balance
- Apoptosis (programmed cell death)
- Aging and longevity

Creatine helps mitochondria in several ways:

- **Buffers ATP production** by supplying phosphate through the phosphocreatine shuttle
- **Reduces mitochondrial stress** by minimizing fluctuations in ADP/ATP ratios
- **Enhances mitochondrial membrane potential**, improving energy efficiency
- **Increases mitochondrial density** in some tissues, particularly muscle

When mitochondrial function falters, chronic fatigue, aging, and diseases like Alzheimer's and Parkinson's become more likely. Creatine's support of these powerhouses is one reason it shows promise in **neurodegenerative conditions and age-related decline**.

3. A Cellular Shield: Antioxidant and Free Radical Scavenger

Every cell in your body faces a constant barrage of threats - from reactive oxygen species (ROS), pollutants, and metabolic byproducts. This oxidative stress is a major driver of:

- Aging
- DNA damage
- Muscle fatigue
- Neurodegeneration
- Chronic diseases like cancer and diabetes

Here's where creatine shines.

Studies have confirmed that creatine acts as both a **direct and indirect antioxidant**:

- It **scavenges harmful radicals** like $ABTS^+$, superoxide (O_2^-), and peroxynitrite ($ONOO^-$)
- It **protects DNA and cell membranes** from oxidative damage
- It **preserves glutathione**, the body's master antioxidant, by reducing its consumption during stress

What makes creatine's antioxidant action unique is that it's **not a traditional vitamin-like antioxidant** (like vitamin C or E). Instead, it helps your **cells manage redox balance internally**, keeping oxidative stress within healthy levels.

This is especially relevant for the brain, where oxidative stress contributes to memory loss, cognitive decline, and mood disorders.

4. Inflammation Control: Calming the Cellular Fire

Inflammation is a double-edged sword: necessary for healing, but destructive when chronic or excessive. In conditions ranging from arthritis and autoimmune disease to cardiovascular dysfunction, **low-grade inflammation erodes tissue function over time**.

Creatine has been shown to **modulate inflammation in several key ways**:

- **Reduces levels of pro-inflammatory cytokines**, such as TNF-α and IL-6
- **Stabilizes endothelial function**, preventing leakage of inflammatory agents into tissues
- **Suppresses microglial overactivation** in the brain (a key feature in neuroinflammation)
- **Improves exercise recovery** by limiting muscle damage and inflammatory response

This anti-inflammatory effect is likely tied to creatine's energy-buffering capabilities. By keeping ATP levels high, cells can maintain membrane integrity and prevent the biochemical cascades that trigger inflammation.

In older adults or those with autoimmune conditions, creatine's anti-inflammatory properties may reduce pain, improve recovery, and **lower the overall inflammatory burden on the body**.

5. Brain Benefits Rooted in Cellular Protection

The brain is one of the most energy-hungry organs in the body. It consumes about **20% of your total energy** - even at rest. During intense thinking, stress, or sleep deprivation, its demand skyrockets.

Creatine provides the brain with:

- **Rapid energy buffering** during cognitive exertion
- **Protection against hypoxia and oxygen deprivation**
- **Support for neurotransmitter synthesis** (including serotonin and dopamine)
- **Defense against neurotoxic stressors**

For example, in sleep-deprived individuals, creatine supplementation has been shown to **improve reaction time and working memory**. In patients with traumatic brain injuries, creatine may **limit the extent of neuronal damage**.

Its ability to enhance **brain resilience**, especially under stress, makes it an emerging candidate for:

- Cognitive enhancement
- Depression treatment
- Traumatic brain injury (TBI) recovery
- Alzheimer's and Parkinson's support

6. Metabolic Health and Glucose Regulation

New research suggests creatine may also play a role in metabolic health, particularly by:

- **Improving glucose uptake into cells**
- **Enhancing insulin sensitivity**

- **Lowering fasting blood glucose and triglycerides**

These effects are likely mediated through creatine's support of **AMP-activated protein kinase (AMPK)**, a key enzyme in metabolic regulation. When energy levels are low, AMPK signals the body to burn fat and increase glucose uptake.

In people with insulin resistance or type 2 diabetes, creatine - especially when paired with exercise - may offer **an additional metabolic edge**.

7. Tissue Hydration and Cell Volume Signaling

Creatine draws water into cells, which leads to:

- **Improved cellular hydration**
- **Better nutrient absorption**
- **Anabolic signaling that promotes protein synthesis**

This is not the "bloating" often misunderstood in popular media. Instead, it's **intracellular water**, which acts as a signal for the cell to **grow, repair, and survive**.

Research shows that increased cell volume can stimulate muscle protein synthesis, inhibit protein breakdown, and even **trigger anti-catabolic pathways**. In essence, well-hydrated cells are healthier cells.

8. Synergistic Healing: Recovery from Injury and Stress

Because creatine supports energy, hydration, inflammation control, and mitochondrial function, it creates the ideal environment for:

- **Wound healing**
- **Muscle repair**

- **Recovery from illness or stress**
- **Adaptation to physical training or injury**

This is especially relevant for:

- Athletes recovering from intense training
- Older adults healing from falls or surgeries
- Individuals dealing with chronic fatigue or stress-related disorders

In these contexts, creatine doesn't just *fuel the system* - it **helps rebuild and protect it**.

Summary: The Invisible Guardian

What we've uncovered in this chapter is a radically different way to see creatine. Not just as a fuel booster, but as a:

- **Cellular stabilizer**
- **Genetic influencer**
- **Anti-inflammatory agent**
- **Antioxidant shield**
- **Mitochondrial ally**

In short, **a quiet molecular guardian that supports the entire cellular ecosystem.**

These "non-energy" effects help explain why creatine seems to benefit such a wide array of systems and diseases. It's not targeting symptoms; it's **fortifying the foundation of cellular function itself**.

Coming Up Next

In Chapter 4: Mind Over Muscle — Creatine's Surprising Impact on the Brain, we'll shift our focus entirely to cognitive and neurological health. You'll learn how creatine improves memory, focus, mood, and brain resilience, and how it may play a role in treating depression, neurodegeneration, and even sleep dysfunction.

Chapter 4 The Brain on Creatine – Cognition, Protection, and Medical Frontiers

From memory and mood to neuroprotection and mental energy

Introduction: Why the Brain Needs More Than Just Willpower

We often think of energy as a physical thing—something our muscles need when we lift, run, or train. But the **brain is the most energy-hungry organ in the human body**, using up to 20% of the body's ATP (adenosine triphosphate) despite comprising only about 2% of body mass.

ATP is the cellular fuel that powers everything from mental focus to emotional regulation. Creatine plays a pivotal role in regenerating ATP—especially during high-demand moments like intense thinking, stress, learning, or sleep deprivation. This has led scientists to explore creatine's powerful—and often underestimated—effects on **brain performance, mood, neuroprotection, and medical conditions**.

In this chapter, we'll explore:

- How creatine affects cognition and mental fatigue
- Its emerging role in mood disorders and neurological protection
- What cutting-edge research reveals about creatine's future in clinical medicine
- How to practically apply creatine for brain-first outcomes

Creatine and Brain Energy: The Cognitive Connection

The brain operates on an "energy budget." When under pressure—think exams, deadlines, or emotional turmoil—it needs rapid ATP turnover. That's where creatine steps in.

What Studies Show:

- **Creatine supplementation has been shown to improve short-term memory, reaction time, and cognitive processing**, especially in tasks requiring sustained mental effort.
- In **vegetarians and vegans**, who typically have lower creatine levels due to dietary absence of meat and fish, the cognitive effects of supplementation are often more pronounced.
- During **sleep deprivation**, creatine may mitigate declines in executive function and working memory, offering a neuroprotective effect.

Creatine doesn't act like caffeine or stimulants; it doesn't **force** wakefulness. Instead, it **supports the brain's bioenergetic stability**, keeping performance high when under pressure.

Creatine and Mood: Depression, Stress, and Resilience

Mental health is tightly linked to energy metabolism. Researchers are now exploring creatine's role in **supporting mood disorders like depression and anxiety**—conditions often marked by mitochondrial dysfunction and low ATP availability.

Clinical Highlights:

- **People with depression often show lower brain phosphocreatine levels**, indicating energy deficits in areas related to emotion regulation.
- Several studies found that **creatine added to antidepressants improves outcomes faster**, especially in women.
- Creatine may also reduce the mental "fog" and lethargy associated with stress, chronic fatigue, or burnout.

In this light, creatine becomes more than a performance supplement—it becomes an **emotional resilience nutrient**, offering fuel to a struggling mind.

Neuroprotection and Aging: Slowing the Slide

As we age, the brain's capacity to generate energy declines, contributing to **cognitive impairment, neurodegenerative disease,** and loss of independence. Creatine's ability to enhance cellular energy has sparked interest in its potential to **slow or prevent age-related cognitive decline.**

Research Is Ongoing in:

- **Alzheimer's disease**
- **Parkinson's disease**
- **Multiple sclerosis (MS)**
- **Traumatic brain injury (TBI)**
- **Stroke recovery**

In animal models and early human trials, creatine has shown the ability to **protect neurons, reduce oxidative stress, and improve mitochondrial function**—all of which are crucial for maintaining a healthy brain as we age.

While creatine is not a cure, its safety profile, affordability, and accessibility make it a promising **adjunct therapy** worth exploring further in medicine.

Creatine at the Medical Frontier: What's Next?

Creatine is currently being studied in medical disciplines far beyond the gym. Here are some of the **emerging frontiers** where creatine could transform care:

1. Mental Health Treatment

- Adjunct therapy for treatment-resistant depression
- Support for bipolar disorder and anxiety
- Mood stabilization during hormonal shifts in women

2. Neurodegenerative Disease Management

- Creatine may slow progression of ALS and Parkinson's (though more human trials are needed)
- Brain volume preservation and protection in early cognitive decline

3. Stroke and Brain Injury Recovery

- Improves cellular energy availability during recovery
- May reduce the extent of post-injury neurological damage

4. Pediatric and Genetic Disorders

- Creatine deficiency syndromes are rare but serious; supplementation can be life-saving
- Research into creatine's impact on **autism spectrum disorders** and **developmental delays** is in early phases

5. Women's Health & Cognition

- Women experience **fluctuations in brain energy needs** across the menstrual cycle, pregnancy, and menopause
- Creatine supplementation has shown **particular benefits in female cognition and emotional balance**, especially when estrogen drops

Practical Applications: Using Creatine for Cognitive and Emotional Support

For brain-related benefits, the dosage and form remain the same as for physical performance:

- **3–5 grams/day of creatine monohydrate**
- No cycling needed; consistent daily use is most effective
- Take with food to aid absorption (especially carbs or insulin-spiking meals)

Who Might Benefit Most?

- **Students & knowledge workers** under mental stress
- **Shift workers & parents** with irregular sleep patterns
- **Older adults** seeking to maintain cognition
- **Anyone with mood imbalances** or stress-related fatigue
- **Women** in perimenopause or postpartum periods

Final Thoughts: One Molecule, Many Minds

The brain's greatest weakness is its energy dependence. When energy fails, thought slows. Mood falters. Memory fades. What creatine offers is not just muscle recovery—it offers **neurological support**, **emotional resilience**, and a new frontier in **preventive brain care**.

As research evolves, it's clear that **creatine has the potential to redefine how we approach brain health in modern medicine**—as both a safeguard for the aging mind and a daily edge for the modern brain.

Summary of Key Takeaways:

- Creatine improves working memory, focus, and cognitive performance
- It may help treat or prevent depression, brain injuries, and cognitive decline
- It supports energy metabolism and mitochondrial function in neurons
- Research is advancing creatine's role in treating neurodegenerative and mood disorders
- Safe for long-term use and highly accessible as a preventive brain supplement

Coming Up Next

In **Chapter 5: Aging Strong — Creatine and the Fight Against Frailty**, we'll turn our attention to how creatine supports the aging body, helping preserve muscle, strength, and independence well into later life. You'll discover how this simple molecule could revolutionize the way we approach healthy aging.

Chapter 5: Aging Strong - Creatine and the Fight Against Frailty

How one molecule is redefining aging, independence, and vitality in older adults

Growing older is inevitable. But growing frail doesn't have to be. As life expectancy increases, the focus of modern healthcare is shifting from simply **adding years to life** to **adding life to years**. In this pursuit, researchers are uncovering a surprisingly powerful ally in the battle against age-related decline: **creatine monohydrate**.

While creatine is often thought of as a supplement for athletes and bodybuilders, research from the past two decades - and particularly the last five years - has spotlighted its unique benefits for aging adults. Creatine can help preserve **muscle mass**, maintain **strength**, improve **balance**, support **cognitive function**, and even **protect bones and metabolic health**.

In this chapter, we explore how creatine is helping older adults **age strong**, remain independent, and push back against the slow creep of frailty.

1. The Physiology of Aging: A Perfect Storm

As we age, our bodies undergo predictable and often destructive changes:

- **Sarcopenia**: the loss of muscle mass and function
- **Dynapenia**: the loss of muscular strength
- **Reduced mitochondrial efficiency**: leading to fatigue
- **Hormonal changes**: reducing anabolic signaling
- **Increased oxidative stress**: accelerating cell damage
- **Cognitive decline**: impacting memory, attention, and processing speed

These changes don't just limit activity - they increase the risk of:

- Falls and fractures
- Hospitalization
- Loss of independence
- Depression and social isolation

In short, aging can be the **perfect storm** for physical and mental decline. But it doesn't have to be. That's where creatine steps in.

2. Creatine + Resistance Training = A Game-Changer for Older Adults

The single most effective strategy to counteract sarcopenia is **resistance training** - but its benefits are **significantly amplified** when paired with creatine supplementation.

Here's what research shows when older adults combine creatine with strength training:

- **Increased total body lean mass** (approx. +1.2 kg on average)
- **Improved upper and lower body strength**
- **Enhanced muscle quality and density**
- **Improved functional performance** (e.g., sit-to-stand test, walking speed)
- **Better balance and reduced fall risk**

One meta-analysis found that older adults who supplemented with creatine while participating in resistance training had **greater gains in strength and mobility** than those who trained without it. And these improvements weren't just statistically significant - they were **clinically meaningful** in real-life outcomes like walking up stairs, getting out of chairs, or preventing falls.

3. Combating Sarcopenia: The Muscle Preserver

Sarcopenia affects nearly **1 in 3 adults over 60**, and its consequences are devastating:

- Difficulty with everyday tasks
- Increased dependence on caregivers
- Higher risk of falls and injury
- Reduced quality of life

Creatine counters sarcopenia through multiple mechanisms:

- **Increases muscle phosphocreatine stores**, enhancing training output
- **Stimulates protein synthesis**, promoting muscle repair and growth
- **Reduces muscle breakdown** during periods of inactivity or illness
- **Enhances satellite cell activity**, aiding in muscle regeneration

Even in older adults not engaging in structured exercise, creatine has been shown to **slow muscle loss**, suggesting its value as a preventive supplement.

4. Supporting Balance, Mobility, and Fall Prevention

Falls are the leading cause of injury-related death in adults over 65. And the risk rises sharply with loss of muscle strength, balance, and coordination.

Creatine can help by:

- **Improving lower-limb power** (critical for climbing stairs or rising from a chair)
- **Enhancing neuromuscular function**, including reaction time
- **Improving proprioception** - the body's sense of its position in space
- **Strengthening muscles involved in posture and gait stability**

By improving these factors, creatine supplementation has been associated with a **reduced risk of falls**, which has cascading benefits for long-term health and independence.

5. Cognitive Protection for Healthy Aging

The benefits of creatine for the aging brain are equally compelling. As covered in Chapter 4, aging leads to:

- **Reduced brain creatine levels**
- **Lower ATP availability**
- **Slower cognitive processing**
- **Increased oxidative stress and neuroinflammation**

Creatine helps reverse these changes by:

- **Improving memory, attention, and mental energy**
- **Supporting mitochondrial health and neuron function**
- **Possibly slowing the onset of neurodegenerative diseases**

Older adults who supplement with creatine may notice:

- **Fewer episodes of "brain fog"**
- **Better memory retention**
- **Improved performance on cognitive tasks**

These benefits are especially pronounced in adults facing metabolic stress (e.g., sleep deprivation, fatigue, or chronic illness), and in those with diets low in meat (such as vegetarians or light meat-eaters).

6. Bone Health: Creatine's Indirect Benefits

While creatine doesn't directly increase **bone mineral density (BMD)** in most studies, it supports bone health in several important ways:

- **Promotes muscle growth**, increasing mechanical load on bones (stimulating bone formation)
- **Improves balance and strength**, reducing the risk of falls and fractures
- **Enhances osteoblast activity** (bone-building cells) in lab studies

A notable pilot study in postmenopausal women found that creatine supplementation **preserved hip BMD** and **slowed bone loss** in the femoral neck region over a two-year period. These findings suggest that creatine may indirectly reduce fracture risk, particularly when combined with resistance exercise.

7. Metabolic Health and Aging

Metabolic diseases like Type 2 diabetes, insulin resistance, and cardiovascular disease increase dramatically with age. Creatine shows promise in modulating several of these conditions:

- **Improves glucose uptake into muscle cells**
- **Lowers fasting blood glucose and triglycerides**
- **May reduce inflammation and oxidative stress**
- **Improves endothelial function (vascular health)**

Aging adults with prediabetes or metabolic syndrome may see **enhanced insulin sensitivity** and **better lipid profiles** after creatine supplementation - especially when combined with exercise.

---

8. Addressing the Aging Appetite: Creatine as Nutritional Insurance

One challenge for older adults is **reduced appetite** and a tendency to eat less protein. This can accelerate muscle loss and nutritional deficiencies.

Creatine offers a **simple, easy-to-digest supplement** that:

- Requires **no cooking or chewing**
- Can be **mixed into water or juice**
- Supports muscle and brain health with **just 3–5 grams per day**

For older adults who can't consume enough protein or calories, creatine serves as **nutritional insurance**, helping prevent or slow the muscle and energy decline associated with undernourishment.

---

9. Is It Safe for Older Adults?

Yes - extensive research confirms that creatine is **safe and well-tolerated** in older adults, including those over 70.

Studies involving thousands of participants have shown:

- No adverse effects on **kidney or liver function** in healthy individuals
- No increase in cardiovascular risk
- Minimal side effects (mild gastrointestinal discomfort in some cases, usually avoidable by splitting doses)

However, caution is advised for individuals with **pre-existing kidney disease**. Regular monitoring and physician guidance are recommended in these cases.

10. Practical Dosing Strategies for Older Adults

Here's how to get started:

- **Loading phase (optional)**: 20 grams/day, divided into 4 doses, for 5–7 days
- **Maintenance**: 3–5 grams/day

For those concerned about bloating or gastrointestinal upset, **skip the loading phase** and go straight to daily dosing. The same results will be achieved over 3–4 weeks.

Creatine is **odorless, tasteless,** and dissolves easily in water, tea, or juice - making it ideal for daily use.

Summary: Redefining Aging with a Simple Supplement

The image of frail, tired aging is becoming obsolete. Science is showing us that **aging strong is possible**, and creatine is one of the most promising tools we have to support that vision.

By maintaining muscle, supporting the brain, aiding balance, and boosting recovery, creatine empowers older adults to:

- Stay mobile and independent
- Reduce fall and fracture risk
- Maintain mental sharpness and mood
- Enjoy a higher quality of life

And all it takes is a **few grams per day**.

Coming Up Next

In **Chapter 6: The Women's Molecule - Creatine Across Female Life Stages**, we'll explore how hormonal changes across menstruation, pregnancy, menopause, and post menopause interact with creatine metabolism - and why **women may be uniquely positioned to benefit from this powerful compound.**

Chapter 6: The Women's Molecule - Creatine Across Female Life Stages

How creatine supports women's health from menstruation to menopause and beyond

Creatine is often associated with men - particularly young, athletic men. Yet this long-standing stereotype is not only outdated, but scientifically inaccurate. In fact, emerging research shows that **women may stand to gain just as much, if not more**, from creatine supplementation than their male counterparts.

Why? Because women generally have **lower baseline creatine levels**, experience **significant hormonal fluctuations**, and face **unique physiological demands** across their lifespan - from menstruation and pregnancy to menopause and aging. These factors all influence **creatine metabolism**, making creatine supplementation not just helpful, but potentially transformative for many women.

This chapter explores the relationship between **female physiology and creatine**, breaking down the benefits at every life stage and offering practical guidance for women seeking better energy, mood, strength, cognition, and resilience.

1. Baseline Differences: Why Women Start at a Creatine Disadvantage

Research consistently shows that **women naturally store less creatine** in their muscles and brains than men - often up to **70–80% less** in some studies. This is due to several factors:

- **Lower dietary intake** (less red meat and fish)
- **Smaller muscle mass**
- **Hormonal regulation** (estrogen influences creatine metabolism)

Because of this, women are **more likely to be creatine-deficient**, especially if they follow a plant-based diet or avoid high-protein foods. This deficiency can contribute to:

- Fatigue
- Reduced physical strength
- Mood fluctuations
- Brain fog and poor memory
- Increased vulnerability to age-related decline

Thankfully, research shows that women **respond exceptionally well** to creatine supplementation - often more dramatically than men, due to the lower starting point.

2. Creatine and the Menstrual Cycle

The menstrual cycle introduces **significant hormonal changes** throughout the month. Estrogen and progesterone, in particular, influence:

- Energy metabolism
- Mood and neurotransmitter levels
- Fluid balance
- Muscle function

These shifts can lead to:

- **Increased fatigue** during the luteal phase
- **Mood instability** and irritability
- **Reduced exercise capacity**
- **Poorer sleep quality**

Creatine can help counteract these effects by:

- Enhancing **brain energy metabolism** during hormonal lows
- Supporting **mood stabilization**
- Improving **sleep duration and quality**
- Buffering **muscle fatigue and recovery**

One study found that creatine improved **short-term memory and reaction time** in women during the luteal phase, when progesterone peaks and estrogen drops - two conditions that can negatively affect cognition.

For women who struggle with PMS or menstrual fatigue, a small daily dose of creatine could become a **valuable tool for managing symptoms** and maintaining performance.

3. Creatine and Pregnancy: A New Frontier

Pregnancy is a metabolically demanding time for both mother and baby. The body experiences:

- Increased energy needs
- Rapid tissue growth
- Heightened oxidative stress
- Fluid and electrolyte shifts

Emerging evidence suggests that **creatine homeostasis is disrupted** during pregnancy - particularly in cases of:

- Preterm birth
- Intrauterine growth restriction (IUGR)
- Preeclampsia
- Maternal hypoxia or stress

In fact, studies show that **57% of pregnant women in the U.S. consume less creatine than recommended**, potentially compromising both maternal and fetal outcomes.

Animal research reveals that **maternal creatine supplementation**:

- Improves **offspring survival**
- Protects **fetal organs** (especially the brain and kidneys)
- Reduces **birth complications** associated with oxygen deprivation

Additionally, maternal creatine status has been correlated with **infant head circumference**, a strong marker for early brain development.

While human trials are still in early stages, the evidence is mounting: **adequate creatine intake may be essential for a healthy pregnancy**, especially in vegetarian or undernourished populations.

4. Perimenopause: Battling the Invisible Decline

Perimenopause - the transitional years leading up to menopause - is a **physiological rollercoaster** marked by:

- Hormonal turbulence
- Muscle and bone loss acceleration
- Sleep disturbances
- Mood instability
- Brain fog and memory issues

It's also a **critical intervention window**. Without nutritional and lifestyle support, many women begin to lose muscle, gain fat, and experience a decline in cognitive and emotional health.

Creatine offers a **multifaceted solution** during this time:

- Helps preserve **lean muscle mass**
- Supports **bone geometry** and strength
- Improves **working memory and cognition**
- May help **stabilize mood** and reduce symptoms of depression
- Enhances **exercise capacity** during fatigue-prone phases

One of creatine's most important benefits during perimenopause is its ability to **delay or attenuate sarcopenia**, which tends to accelerate as estrogen levels fall.

Combined with resistance training, creatine acts as a **buffer against the biological turbulence** of this life stage.

5. Postmenopause: Staying Strong, Sharp, and Independent

After menopause, women experience:

- **Estrogen withdrawal**
- **Accelerated muscle and bone loss**
- **Greater insulin resistance**
- **Cognitive decline risk**
- **Increased inflammation and oxidative stress**

This can lead to frailty, osteoporosis, mobility loss, and even cognitive disorders like Alzheimer's.

Creatine steps in as a **lifeline**:

- Builds and preserves **muscle mass and strength**
- Enhances **bone-loading force** through improved muscular output
- Protects **neuronal health** and may improve memory
- May improve **insulin sensitivity** and reduce metabolic disease risk

- Supports **daily energy** and reduces **chronic fatigue**

Studies show that postmenopausal women taking creatine, especially when paired with resistance training, see significant improvements in:

- **Muscle function**
- **Walking speed**
- **Grip strength**
- **Balance and reaction time**

In fact, creatine is one of the **few supplements clinically shown** to improve both **physical and cognitive resilience** in postmenopausal women.

6. Mental Health and Mood: A Gendered Response

Depression and anxiety affect women **twice as often** as men, and hormonal fluctuations are a major contributing factor.

Creatine shows particular promise for women's mental health:

- Enhances **serotonin and dopamine production**
- Improves **brain energy balance**
- Augments response to **antidepressant therapy**
- Reduces **perceived fatigue and mental burnout**

Several studies have shown that women with **major depressive disorder** respond **more rapidly and strongly** to antidepressant therapy when creatine is added to the treatment plan. This may be due to **female-specific creatine kinetics**, which alter how creatine is metabolized in the brain.

The implications? Creatine could become a **key adjunct** in treating hormone-related mood disorders like PMDD, postpartum depression, and menopausal mood shifts.

7. Dosing for Women: What Works Best?

Because of lower baseline creatine levels and different body compositions, women may respond better to **lower or moderate doses** over time.

Recommended dosing strategies:

- **Daily use**: 3–5 grams/day
- **No loading phase needed** for most women
- For brain-related outcomes (e.g., mood or memory): consider **5–10 grams/day**, especially during stress or hormonal change
- During pregnancy or perimenopause: **consult a physician** for personalized guidance

Creatine can be easily added to:

- Water, juice, or tea
- Protein shakes
- Yogurt or oatmeal

There's **no need to cycle** on and off. Long-term daily use is safe for healthy women.

8. Breaking the Myth: "Creatine Will Make Me Bulky"

Let's be clear: **creatine does not masculinize women**.

It:

- Does **not increase testosterone**
- Does **not cause excessive weight gain**

- Does **not cause bloating** when used correctly

What it does do is:

- Increase **cellular hydration**
- Support **muscle tone and definition**
- Help maintain a **leaner body composition**

Any small increase in weight is typically due to **intracellular water retention**, not fat or "bulk." And this water retention is **functional and beneficial**, improving muscle efficiency and nutrient flow.

Creatine is **body-positive**, not body-altering.

Summary: A Supplement for Every Stage

From first period to postmenopause, creatine is a uniquely supportive supplement for women. It:

- Compensates for low baseline levels
- Buffers hormonal fluctuations
- Supports both brain and body health
- Offers energy, mood, and cognitive enhancement
- Helps build strength and resilience throughout life

It's time to retire the myth that creatine is "for men" and embrace its role as a **critical micronutrient for female well-being**.

Coming Up Next

In **Chapter 7: Creatine for the Mindful Eater - Benefits for Vegans and Vegetarians**, we'll examine how plant-based eaters - who consume little to no creatine through diet - respond more dramatically to supplementation, and how this can support performance, cognition, and nutritional balance.

Chapter 7: Creatine for the Mindful Eater - Benefits for Vegans and Vegetarians

Unlocking the hidden power of creatine for those who eat plant-based

In the age of conscious eating, plant-based diets are booming. Whether for ethical, environmental, or health reasons, millions are shifting toward vegetarian and vegan lifestyles. While this shift offers many well-documented benefits - reduced risk of cardiovascular disease, lower inflammation, and improved gut health - it also comes with certain nutritional trade-offs.

One of the most significant and often overlooked of these trade-offs is **creatine deficiency**.

Unlike vitamins or minerals, creatine isn't typically listed on a nutrition label. It doesn't have a daily recommended intake, and it's not something you can "eyeball" in your diet. But if you're not eating animal products, chances are you're not getting much - if any - of this critical nutrient.

This chapter explores how plant-based eaters can harness the science of creatine to **support cognition, improve exercise performance, boost mood**, and safeguard long-term health - without compromising their dietary values.

1. What Is Creatine, and Why Are Vegans Low in It?

Creatine is a **nitrogenous organic compound** synthesized in the body from amino acids (arginine, glycine, and methionine). While the body can produce about 1–2 grams per day, this is typically **not enough to saturate muscle and brain stores**, especially under physical or mental stress.

The **primary dietary sources** of creatine are:

- Red meat
- Poultry
- Fish
- Eggs (to a much lesser extent)

These are foods that **vegans and most vegetarians exclude**. As a result:

- **Vegans often have 10–30% lower muscle creatine levels**
- **Brain creatine levels may also be lower**, though harder to measure directly
- **Total body creatine stores are reduced**, impairing high-energy functions

This deficiency isn't obvious - it doesn't show up on blood tests or cause symptoms overnight. But over time, it can contribute to:

- **Lower strength and endurance**
- **Slower recovery**
- **Increased mental fatigue**
- **Cognitive "fogginess"**
- **Greater risk of muscle and bone loss with age**

Fortunately, creatine supplementation can **fully restore and even optimize** these stores.

2. The Plant-Based Performance Gap - and How to Fix It

A common observation among plant-based athletes and fitness enthusiasts is a **slight underperformance in high-intensity, short-duration efforts**. This isn't due to protein deficiency - it's often due to **reduced creatine availability**.

Studies consistently show that when vegans and vegetarians **supplement with creatine**, they experience:

- **Greater increases in strength**
- **More lean muscle gains**
- **Improved sprint and power output**
- **Enhanced endurance during interval training**

One landmark study found that vegetarian participants experienced **twice the improvement in high-intensity cycling performance** compared to omnivores when supplemented with creatine.

Why? Because their muscles were **farther from saturation** - so the supplementation had a **bigger impact**.

In short, plant-based diets make creatine supplementation **more necessary and more effective.**

3. Cognitive Enhancement: Creatine for the Vegan Brain

Creatine isn't just about muscles - it's crucial for the brain, too.

The brain demands a **constant, high supply of ATP** to maintain focus, memory, problem-solving, and emotional regulation. And like muscle, the brain relies on **creatine-phosphocreatine buffering** to meet sudden energy demands.

For vegans and vegetarians, this is especially important because:

- **Lower brain creatine** may impair cognitive resilience under stress
- **Memory and executive function** may decline more quickly under sleep deprivation or multitasking
- **Mental fatigue** may occur sooner during prolonged work or study

In one double-blind study, vegetarian participants who took creatine showed:

- **Significant improvements in working memory**
- **Faster reaction times**
- **Better performance on IQ-type tasks**
- **Reduced perceived fatigue**

For students, professionals, and anyone facing high cognitive demands, creatine offers a **safe, ethical, and potent mental performance enhancer**.

4. Creatine and Mood: Mental Health in Plant-Based Diets

Although plant-based diets have many mental health benefits - thanks to higher fiber, antioxidants, and phytonutrients - they may inadvertently limit some compounds critical to **neurotransmitter synthesis and brain function**, such as:

- Creatine
- Vitamin B12
- Iron
- Choline
- DHA (from omega-3)

This may partly explain why some studies have found **higher rates of depression and anxiety** in strictly vegan populations (though data is mixed and confounded by lifestyle factors).

Creatine helps bridge this gap by:

- Supporting **serotonin and dopamine metabolism**
- Enhancing **brain energy balance**
- Reducing **oxidative and inflammatory stress** in neurons

- Potentially **improving response to antidepressants**

Several trials, especially in women and under high-stress conditions, show that creatine supplementation leads to:

- **Improved mood**
- **Reduced symptoms of depression**
- **Lower perceived stress and burnout**

This makes creatine an **important safeguard** for those on plant-based diets facing high cognitive or emotional demands.

5. Creatine and Bone Health in Meat-Free Diets

Vegetarians and vegans tend to have **lower bone mineral density (BMD)** than omnivores, likely due to:

- Reduced calcium and vitamin D intake
- Lower dietary protein
- Fewer anabolic stimuli from muscle mass and loading
- Lower creatine levels

While creatine does not directly increase BMD, it:

- Enhances **muscle mass**, which loads bones through movement
- Improves **balance and strength**, reducing fall risk
- Supports **osteoblast (bone-forming cell) metabolism** in lab models

Combined with resistance training, creatine can serve as an **indirect yet powerful tool** for improving skeletal strength in plant-based eaters.

6. Overcoming the Stigma: "Natural" Supplements for Natural Diets

Some plant-based purists may hesitate to use creatine, seeing it as a "synthetic" or "unnatural" supplement. But here's what's important to know:

- **Creatine monohydrate is vegan**: Most high-quality supplements today are synthesized from sarcosine and cyanamide - no animal ingredients involved.
- **It mimics what's found in food**: Supplementation simply replaces what an omnivore might get from meat.
- **It is scientifically safe and effective**: Backed by decades of clinical trials.

Far from being unnatural, creatine may be **the most natural thing missing** from a plant-based lifestyle - and one of the easiest to restore.

7. Dosing Recommendations for Vegans and Vegetarians

Because baseline levels are lower, plant-based individuals may benefit from:

- **Loading phase**: 20 grams/day for 5–7 days (optional)
- **Maintenance**: 3–5 grams/day
- For brain benefits or mental health: **5–10 grams/day**, depending on stress or activity level

Creatine monohydrate is best taken:

- With a meal (insulin enhances uptake)
- Consistently, at the same time each day
- Mixed with juice, smoothies, or plant-based protein shakes

There's no need to "cycle off." Continuous use is safe and supports sustained benefits.

8. Real-World Examples: How Plant-Based People Use Creatine

- **Emma, 28** – A vegan personal trainer: "Creatine helped me finally break through my plateau. My lifts improved, and I felt more energetic between sets."
- **Carlos, 42** – A vegetarian software engineer: "I started creatine to fight brain fog during crunch weeks. Within two weeks, I noticed I could focus longer without burning out."
- **Lila, 34** – A yoga instructor and wellness coach: "I was skeptical, but after researching the science, I started supplementing. My recovery improved, and I feel sharper and more balanced emotionally."

These stories highlight what science is now confirming: **creatine isn't just for bodybuilders. It's for mindful eaters who want to protect and optimize their energy, cognition, and strength.**

Summary: A Missing Piece of the Plant-Based Puzzle

If you eat a vegetarian or vegan diet, you may be:

- Health-conscious
- Ethically motivated
- Environmentally aware

But you may also be missing one of the **key nutrients** that supports full-body wellness. Creatine offers:

- **Strength for your workouts**
- **Focus for your work**
- **Resilience for your nervous system**
- **Longevity for your muscles and bones**

All without compromising your values.

Supplementing with creatine is not a step back from your plant-based journey - it's a **step forward toward a stronger, smarter, and more energized you.**

Coming Up Next

In **Chapter 8: Bones of Steel - Creatine's Role in Skeletal Strength,** we'll dig deeper into how creatine supports bone health - not just through density, but through geometry, force absorption, and fracture protection. You'll learn how this molecule contributes to long-term skeletal integrity and how it pairs with exercise to keep you standing tall.

Chapter 8: Bones of Steel - Creatine's Role in Skeletal Strength

How creatine strengthens the body's structural foundation from the inside out

When we think of bones, we usually picture dense, rigid structures - support beams that hold our bodies upright. But bones are far from static. They are dynamic, metabolically active tissues constantly undergoing remodeling. They respond to hormones, mechanical forces, and nutritional inputs. And while nutrients like calcium and vitamin D get the spotlight for bone health, research now reveals that **creatine may also play a critical and overlooked role**.

In this chapter, we'll explore how creatine helps protect your skeletal system - not just by improving bone density, but by enhancing the **muscle-bone interface**, reducing **fracture risk**, supporting **bone geometry**, and improving **bone cell metabolism**.

It turns out that creatine may be just as important for bones as it is for biceps.

1. Bones and Muscles: A Symbiotic Relationship

Bones and muscles don't operate in isolation. They are **deeply interconnected**, with each influencing the other:

- Muscles generate **force** that stimulates bone remodeling.
- Bones respond to this force by **increasing density, thickness, and strength**.
- Weak muscles mean **less mechanical loading** on bones, accelerating bone loss.

This interaction is governed by **Wolff's Law,** which states that bones adapt to the loads placed upon them.

Creatine enters the picture by:

- Enhancing **muscle size and strength**
- Increasing **mechanical force exerted on bones**
- Improving **neuromuscular coordination and balance**

Together, these effects **stimulate bone growth and reduce fall-related fracture risk** - a critical issue in aging populations.

2. Bone Health Beyond Density: The Geometry Factor

When most people think of strong bones, they think of **bone mineral density (BMD)** - often measured by DEXA scans. And while BMD is important, it's only one piece of the puzzle. Bones also rely on:

- **Geometry** (e.g., thickness, cross-sectional area)
- **Microarchitecture**
- **Material quality and resilience to bending or torsion**

Emerging research shows that **creatine may positively influence bone geometry**, particularly in weight-bearing bones like the femur and hip.

One study found that older women supplementing with creatine during a one-year resistance training program experienced:

- **Preserved hip BMD**
- **Improved femoral geometry**
- **Reduced femoral neck bone loss over two years**

These changes matter. Even small improvements in structure can reduce fracture risk by improving **impact resistance**.

3. Creatine and Bone Cells: The Osteoblast Connection

Bone is constantly remodeled by two key cells:

- **Osteoblasts** – build new bone
- **Osteoclasts** – break down bone

Osteoblasts are **energy-hungry** cells. They require ATP to:

- Synthesize bone matrix proteins
- Transport minerals
- Signal other bone cells

Creatine supports these processes by:

- Enhancing **ATP availability via the phosphocreatine system**
- Stimulating **osteoblast differentiation and activity**
- Promoting **mineralization** (laying down calcium and phosphate)

In vitro studies (lab models) show that creatine:

- Increases osteoblast metabolic rate
- Improves their ability to form strong bone tissue
- Reduces markers of **bone resorption** (breakdown)

This suggests that creatine doesn't just help muscles push on bones - it helps **build the bones themselves.**

4. Fracture Prevention: A Functional Perspective

Each year, millions of older adults suffer hip fractures - a leading cause of disability, hospitalizations, and even mortality. The best fracture prevention strategy isn't just denser bones; it's a combination of:

- **Stronger muscles**
- **Faster reflexes**
- **Better balance**
- **More coordinated movement**

Creatine contributes to all of these by:

- Improving **leg strength and power**
- Enhancing **neuromuscular function**
- Reducing **fall frequency**
- Supporting **postural stability**

For older adults, especially women at high risk for osteoporosis, creatine is not just a **bone support supplement** - it's a **mobility and safety strategy**.

5. Synergy with Resistance Training

As with many of creatine's benefits, the effects on bone are **amplified when paired with resistance training**.

Here's how it works:

- Resistance training stresses both muscles and bones.
- Creatine boosts **training volume and intensity**.
- Stronger muscles exert more force on bones, promoting **bone modeling**.

- Repeated loading leads to **increased bone strength** and reduced fragility.

Studies have shown that combining resistance training and creatine leads to:

- **Greater improvements in muscle and bone strength**
- **Enhanced mobility and functional performance**
- **Better outcomes than training alone**

Even in women over 60 and postmenopausal adults, the combination of strength training + creatine **slows bone loss** and improves quality of life.

6. Bone Health Across the Lifespan

While bone decline is typically associated with aging, the groundwork for skeletal strength is laid much earlier - **especially in adolescence and early adulthood**.

Here's how creatine benefits each life stage:

Adolescents & Young Adults

- Bone mass accrues rapidly during puberty.
- Creatine may support **optimal bone formation** when combined with sports and activity.
- Ideal for **athletic young women**, especially those with low energy availability.

Premenopausal Women

- Creatine may help **reduce bone turnover**, especially during menstrual cycles.

- May be protective in women with low dietary protein or low estrogen levels.

Postmenopausal Women

- Most at risk for osteoporosis due to estrogen decline.
- Creatine + resistance training = **a powerful defense** against age-related bone loss.

Older Adults

- At risk for falls and fractures.
- Creatine improves **strength, balance, and bone geometry** - supporting skeletal resilience.

In every stage, creatine contributes not only to **bone strength** but to the **muscular scaffolding** that supports and protects bones.

7. Dosing for Bone Benefits

There's no bone-specific "creatine dose," but research suggests:

- **3–5 grams/day** is sufficient for long-term use
- **No loading phase is required**, especially in older adults
- When aiming for cognitive or metabolic synergy, **5–10 grams/day** may offer added benefit

Consistency is key. Bone remodeling is a **slow process**, and benefits may take **months to accumulate**. Pairing creatine with **weight-bearing exercise** (walking, squats, lunges, resistance bands) is essential for maximal results.

8. Safety and Side Notes

Creatine is safe for long-term use in bone-focused populations, including:

- **Postmenopausal women**
- **Older adults with no kidney disease**
- **Individuals with low BMD or osteopenia**

There is no evidence that creatine interferes with:

- Calcium absorption
- Vitamin D metabolism
- Hormonal balance (unlike some osteoporosis drugs)

And unlike bisphosphonates or hormone therapy, creatine:

- Is **non-pharmaceutical**
- Has **no serious side effects**
- Supports **multiple body systems at once**

Summary: Building Bones from the Bottom Up

Bone health is more than taking calcium pills or avoiding falls. It's about building a **strong foundation through muscular power, cellular energy, and consistent movement**.

Creatine supports this mission by:

- Enhancing **muscle-driven bone loading**
- Stimulating **bone cell function**
- Improving **balance and mobility**
- Reducing **fall and fracture risk**

It's a foundational supplement not just for athletes, but for anyone who wants to **stand tall for life**.

Coming Up Next

In **Chapter 9: Heart and Metabolism - Creatine's Hidden Cardiovascular Potential**, we'll dive into the exciting and still-emerging world of creatine's impact on vascular health, blood sugar regulation, triglycerides, and metabolic resilience. You'll learn how creatine might protect not just your muscles - but your heart.

Chapter 9: Heart and Metabolism - Creatine's Hidden Cardiovascular Potential

How creatine supports vascular health, blood sugar balance, and metabolic resilience

If someone handed you a compound that could support your heart, balance your blood sugar, lower triglycerides, and fight inflammation - most people wouldn't guess creatine. But perhaps they should.

While creatine is best known for boosting muscle performance, a growing body of research is revealing its **hidden potential in cardiovascular and metabolic health**. From improving blood vessel elasticity to enhancing glucose metabolism and reducing harmful fats in the blood, creatine appears to do far more than fuel your workouts. It may help **protect your most vital organ systems** - especially as you age.

This chapter will uncover how creatine supports your heart, arteries, blood sugar, and metabolic stability, offering a **simple but powerful intervention** in the fight against chronic disease.

---

1. A Shift in Focus: From Strength to Systemic Health

In recent years, chronic diseases like cardiovascular disease (CVD), Type 2 diabetes, and metabolic syndrome have become global health crises. These conditions share a common thread:

- **Oxidative stress**
- **Chronic inflammation**
- **Poor glucose control**
- **Vascular dysfunction**

What's remarkable is that creatine - long relegated to gym culture - is now being studied as a **low-cost, low-risk intervention** for these major health concerns. Why? Because it works at the level of **cellular energy, antioxidant defense, and inflammation regulation** - mechanisms that underpin virtually all metabolic functions.

Let's examine how creatine supports each of these areas.

2. Vascular Health: Supporting Arteries and Blood Flow

A healthy cardiovascular system depends on flexible blood vessels, efficient blood flow, and strong endothelial function (the lining of your blood vessels). As we age, or in the presence of inflammation, these vessels become stiff and dysfunctional, increasing the risk of:

- High blood pressure
- Atherosclerosis
- Stroke and heart attack

Preliminary research shows that creatine may improve vascular health by:

- Enhancing **flow-mediated dilation (FMD%)** - a measure of how well arteries expand in response to blood flow
- Supporting **microvascular reperfusion** - blood flow into tiny capillaries after stress or constriction
- Protecting **endothelial cells** from oxidative damage

In one pilot study, older adults taking creatine experienced a **1.22% increase in FMD%** - a modest-sounding improvement that translates into a **13% decrease in future cardiovascular event risk**.

The proposed mechanisms include:

- **Increased nitric oxide availability**
- **Reduction in oxidative radicals** that damage blood vessels
- **Improved ATP delivery to endothelial cells**

These benefits suggest creatine could support both **macrovascular health (arteries)** and **microvascular health (capillaries)** - critical for organs like the brain, heart, kidneys, and eyes.

---

3. Blood Sugar Regulation: Creatine and Glucose Metabolism

Creatine may also support **healthy blood glucose control**, making it a potentially valuable tool for people with:

- Prediabetes
- Type 2 diabetes
- Metabolic syndrome
- Insulin resistance (common in aging and obesity)

In clinical trials, creatine supplementation:

- Reduced **fasting blood glucose** from prediabetic to healthy levels
- Improved **glucose uptake into muscle tissue**, especially when combined with exercise
- Enhanced **glycogen storage** (muscle energy reserve) after carbohydrate intake

How does it work?

The muscle is the **largest site of glucose disposal in the body**. Creatine helps:

- Increase **muscle volume and energy demand**
- Activate **GLUT-4 transporters**, which shuttle glucose into cells
- Improve **insulin signaling pathways**

This means more glucose goes **into your muscles** for fuel and storage, rather than remaining elevated in your bloodstream.

For individuals with sedentary lifestyles or those struggling with blood sugar fluctuations, creatine (especially when paired with walking or resistance training) may offer a **simple, effective strategy for glycemic control**.

4. Lipid Profile Improvements: Reducing Triglycerides and Fat Load

High triglycerides are a known risk factor for heart disease, stroke, and metabolic disorders. In addition to glucose regulation, creatine supplementation has been associated with:

- **Reduced fasting triglyceride levels**
- Improved **lipid metabolism**
- Possibly enhanced **fat oxidation during exercise**

Although more studies are needed to confirm long-term benefits, early evidence suggests that creatine supports a **healthier blood lipid profile** - especially in older adults or those with metabolic syndrome.

5. Anti-Inflammatory and Antioxidant Properties

Chronic inflammation and oxidative stress are at the core of nearly every chronic illness, including:

- Atherosclerosis
- Diabetes
- Obesity
- Autoimmune conditions

Creatine combats these through:

- **Antioxidant activity**: Scavenging reactive oxygen species like superoxide and peroxynitrite
- **Protecting mitochondrial function**, reducing free radical generation at the source
- **Reducing pro-inflammatory cytokines**, such as TNF-alpha and IL-6
- **Suppressing endothelial permeability**, which reduces vascular inflammation

These effects help maintain **vascular integrity**, preserve **insulin sensitivity**, and protect against **DNA and protein damage** - all essential for long-term cardiovascular and metabolic health.

6. Homocysteine Reduction: A Hidden Cardiovascular Benefit?

Homocysteine is an amino acid that, when elevated, is associated with increased risk of:

- Heart disease
- Stroke
- Blood clots
- Cognitive decline

The body uses **S-adenosylmethionine (SAMe)** to synthesize creatine naturally. When you supplement with creatine, you **reduce the body's demand for SAMe**, thereby **sparing methyl groups** and potentially lowering homocysteine production.

While human trials are still limited, animal models suggest that creatine supplementation **reduces homocysteine levels**, particularly in the context of kidney disease or impaired methylation pathways. This could offer an

indirect cardioprotective benefit, especially for people with B-vitamin deficiencies or elevated homocysteine.

7. Creatine in Type 2 Diabetes and Metabolic Syndrome

Type 2 diabetes is more than high blood sugar - it's a complex disorder involving:

- **Insulin resistance**
- **Mitochondrial dysfunction**
- **Increased oxidative stress**
- **Chronic inflammation**

Creatine addresses each of these by:

- Enhancing **mitochondrial energy production**
- Improving **glucose clearance**
- Supporting **muscle insulin sensitivity**
- Reducing **inflammatory signaling**

Preliminary studies have shown that people with insulin resistance or Type 2 diabetes may respond positively to creatine, particularly when **paired with aerobic or resistance exercise**.

In short: **creatine helps muscles "soak up" more sugar and fat**, reducing the burden on your bloodstream and your pancreas.

8. Practical Use: Creatine for Heart and Metabolic Health

If you're interested in using creatine for cardiovascular or metabolic benefits, here's what you need to know:

Recommended Dosing:

- **Start with 3–5 grams/day**
- **No need to load**, unless also using for athletic purposes
- For brain and vascular goals: **5–10 grams/day** may provide more benefit
- Take with a meal to enhance insulin-mediated uptake

Who Benefits Most:

- Adults over 40
- People with family history of CVD or diabetes
- Individuals with high triglycerides or blood pressure
- Sedentary people looking to begin an exercise program
- Those on plant-based or low-protein diets

Combine With:

- **Exercise**, especially walking or resistance training
- **Anti-inflammatory diets** (e.g., Mediterranean or plant-based)
- **Omega-3 fatty acids** and **magnesium** for synergistic cardiovascular support

9. Addressing Concerns: Is It Safe for the Heart?

Yes. Clinical studies and long-term trials show that creatine is:

- **Safe for healthy individuals**, including older adults
- **Well-tolerated** even at higher doses
- **Non-stimulatory**, making it safe for those with hypertension or arrhythmias

That said, individuals with **pre-existing kidney disease** or **on certain medications** (e.g., nephrotoxic drugs or diuretics) should consult their physician before supplementing.

Summary: From Muscle to Metabolism

Creatine is rapidly evolving from a niche sports supplement into a **versatile, system-wide health optimizer**. When it comes to heart and metabolic health, its benefits are clear:

- **Improves blood flow and vascular flexibility**
- **Lowers blood glucose and triglycerides**
- **Supports insulin sensitivity and mitochondrial function**
- **Reduces oxidative stress and inflammation**

Whether you're looking to **prevent disease, enhance exercise**, or simply **age more gracefully**, creatine provides a compelling, research-backed solution.

Coming Up Next

In **Chapter 10: Hope for the Chronically Ill — Creatine as a Therapeutic Ally**, we'll explore how creatine is being investigated as a supportive therapy for clinical conditions ranging from muscular dystrophies to arthritis, fibromyalgia, and even brain injury recovery. You'll discover how this humble molecule could soon play a role in hospitals, not just gyms.

Chapter 10: Hope for the Chronically Ill - Creatine as a Therapeutic Ally

Supporting healing, energy, and function across clinical conditions

When we think of dietary supplements used in medicine, we often imagine vitamins and minerals - iron for anemia, vitamin D for bone health, omega-3s for heart protection. But increasingly, one compound is stepping out of the gym and into the clinic: **creatine monohydrate**.

From muscle-wasting disorders to brain injuries, from chronic fatigue to rheumatic diseases, creatine is being investigated as a **therapeutic adjunct** - a low-cost, well-tolerated supplement that can support recovery, energy metabolism, and quality of life in people facing long-term health challenges.

This chapter explores creatine's growing role as a **clinically relevant tool** - not as a miracle cure, but as a **biological ally** that helps the body function better under stress, disease, and healing.

---

1. Creatine in Muscular Dystrophy and Neuromuscular Disorders

Muscular dystrophies (MD) and myopathies are genetic disorders characterized by:

- Progressive **muscle wasting**
- Loss of **functional mobility**
- **Fatigue**, weakness, and reduced endurance

In these conditions, the muscle's ability to store and use energy is compromised - and this is where creatine shines.

What the research shows:

- Supplementation can **increase muscle strength**
- Improves **functional performance**, such as walking distance or stair climbing
- Helps **delay fatigue**
- Reduces **muscle damage** during daily activities

Children and adults with **Duchenne MD**, **Becker MD**, or **inflammatory myopathies** have shown measurable improvements in strength and daily function when creatine is added to their care plan.

While not curative, creatine provides a **practical and affordable option** to support better quality of life.

---

2. Chronic Fatigue Syndrome (CFS) and Fibromyalgia

CFS and fibromyalgia are complex, often debilitating syndromes involving:

- Profound fatigue
- Cognitive dysfunction ("brain fog")
- Muscle pain and sensitivity
- Sleep disturbances

These conditions are frequently linked to **mitochondrial dysfunction, impaired energy metabolism**, and **neuroinflammation** - areas where creatine exerts direct effects.

Potential benefits of creatine in CFS/Fibromyalgia:

- Improves **brain and muscle ATP production**
- Reduces **perceived exertion and fatigue**
- Enhances **recovery after activity**

- May reduce **pain sensitivity** through neuroprotective mechanisms

While studies are still limited, early evidence and patient reports suggest creatine can serve as an **energy support buffer**, especially when combined with gentle exercise, pacing, and anti-inflammatory strategies.

3. Creatine in Arthritis and Rheumatic Conditions

Osteoarthritis (OA), rheumatoid arthritis (RA), and fibromyalgia all involve:

- **Joint pain**
- **Muscle weakness**
- **Inflammation**
- **Reduced physical activity**

Creatine can help:

- Increase **muscle strength** surrounding affected joints
- Improve **function and mobility**, making exercise more feasible
- Reduce **inflammatory markers**, such as TNF-α and CRP
- Support **recovery from exercise or flare-ups**

In individuals with **knee osteoarthritis**, for example, creatine has been shown to:

- Improve **quadriceps strength**
- Enhance **gait performance**
- Reduce **stiffness and fatigue**

These improvements translate into **better stair climbing, walking, and pain management** - without pharmaceutical side effects.

4. Brain Injury and Traumatic Neurological Events

Creatine's role in **neuroprotection** makes it an exciting candidate for treating:

- **Traumatic brain injury (TBI)**
- **Concussions**
- **Stroke recovery**
- **Hypoxic-ischemic brain injury** (especially in infants or during childbirth)

When the brain is injured, there is often:

- **ATP depletion**
- **Cellular swelling and acidosis**
- **Inflammatory cascade**
- **Oxidative damage**

Creatine addresses all four by:

- Rapidly restoring **brain ATP**
- Reducing **cellular swelling and calcium overload**
- Acting as an **antioxidant**
- Preserving **mitochondrial function**

Clinical findings:

- In children with TBI, creatine reduced **hospital stay lengths**, **headache frequency**, and **vomiting**
- In adults, creatine may aid **cognitive recovery and motor function**, especially when taken prophylactically

While more research is needed, the safety and neuroprotective potential of creatine make it a **promising addition to brain injury recovery protocols**.

5. Cardiovascular and Kidney Disease

While creatine is generally safe for most people, its role in **clinical populations with organ dysfunction** is more nuanced.

In cardiovascular disease:

- Creatine may improve **vascular function**, as discussed in Chapter 9
- Helps enhance **exercise tolerance**, which is critical in cardiac rehab
- May protect against **oxidative stress** and improve **blood flow** during activity

In kidney disease:

- Creatine does **not harm kidney function in healthy individuals**
- But in people with **pre-existing kidney impairment**, creatine should be used with caution
- There is early evidence (from animal models) that creatine **might** help manage **uremic complications** and **homocysteine levels**, but human data is limited

Conclusion: Creatine is potentially valuable in early-stage or well-managed cardiovascular disease - but **requires medical supervision in renal-compromised individuals**.

6. Type 2 Diabetes and Insulin Resistance

Type 2 diabetes is a major global health issue. As discussed in Chapter 9, creatine helps:

- Improve **glucose uptake**
- Support **muscle glycogen storage**
- Enhance **training capacity** in diabetic individuals

New research shows that **creatine may act synergistically with exercise** to:

- Improve **insulin sensitivity**
- Lower **fasting blood sugar**
- Reduce **oxidative stress** in pancreatic beta cells

For diabetics engaging in exercise therapy or rehab, creatine could **magnify the effects of training** and **protect metabolic tissues** from damage.

7. Depression and Mental Health Disorders

Creatine's benefits in mood disorders have already been touched on in previous chapters, but in clinical populations, the relevance is growing.

Major depressive disorder (MDD), bipolar disorder, and anxiety disorders often involve:

- **Mitochondrial dysfunction**
- **Neuroinflammation**
- **Neurotransmitter imbalance**

Creatine addresses these issues by:

- Supporting **brain energy metabolism**
- Enhancing **serotonin and dopamine pathways**
- Increasing **response rates to SSRI medications**

In one study, women with depression who added **5 grams of creatine daily** to their SSRI regimen experienced **faster and more profound mood improvements** than those on antidepressants alone.

These findings suggest creatine may become a **standard adjunct in psychiatric care**, particularly in cases of **treatment-resistant depression**.

8. Cancer and Cachexia

Cancer patients undergoing treatment often experience **cachexia** - a severe form of muscle wasting and weight loss due to:

- Inflammation
- Nutritional deficiencies
- Chemotherapy side effects

While not a cure, creatine has shown potential to:

- **Preserve muscle mass**
- Improve **strength and energy**
- Support **appetite and daily function**

These benefits are most likely when creatine is combined with:

- **Resistance or mobility exercises**
- **Nutritional support**
- **Anti-inflammatory interventions**

Given its excellent safety profile, creatine may soon be more widely adopted in **oncology rehabilitation programs**.

9. Clinical Use Guidelines and Considerations

Dosing for therapeutic support:

- **3–5 grams/day** is sufficient for most chronic conditions
- **5–10 grams/day** may be used for cognitive or neuroprotective goals
- For children or underweight individuals: adjust to **0.1 g/kg body weight**

Administration tips:

- Can be added to **water, juice, or smoothies**
- Should be taken **daily**, preferably with meals
- Is **safe for long-term use**, even in older adults

Monitoring:

- Individuals with **renal impairment** should consult their doctor and be monitored regularly
- Those on multiple medications (e.g., diuretics, nephrotoxic drugs) should check for potential interactions

---

Summary: A Low-Risk, High-Impact Adjunct to Care

Creatine is not a replacement for medications or medical care - but it **amplifies healing and resilience** across many chronic conditions. It:

- Restores **cellular energy**
- Supports **physical strength**
- Protects **neuronal and mitochondrial function**
- Improves **cognition and mental health**
- Enhances **recovery, quality of life, and independence**

For clinicians, caregivers, and patients alike, creatine represents a **scientifically grounded, patient-friendly supplement** that bridges the gap between fitness and medicine.

In **Chapter 11: Safety First - Debunking Myths and Understanding the Risks**, we'll take a deep dive into creatine's safety profile, explore common misconceptions, and look at how this supplement has earned its reputation as one of the most thoroughly tested and well-tolerated nutritional aids in existence.

Chapter 11: Safety First - Debunking Myths and Understanding the Risks

What every consumer, clinician, and caregiver should know about creatine's safety profile

With all the powerful benefits discussed in previous chapters - muscle building, cognitive enhancement, cardiovascular support, and therapeutic applications - one question inevitably surfaces:

Is creatine safe?

Few supplements have been studied as extensively as creatine monohydrate. Over **1,000 peer-reviewed studies** have been conducted on creatine's efficacy, side effects, dosing, and long-term use. The overwhelming consensus is clear: **creatine is not only effective - it is among the safest supplements available** when used appropriately.

Yet despite the science, creatine continues to be clouded by **myths and misinformation**. In this chapter, we'll separate fact from fiction, explore real safety data, clarify who should or shouldn't use it, and provide clear, responsible guidelines for confident, long-term use.

1. The Safety Record: What the Science Says

Creatine has been in widespread use for **over 30 years**, with studies including:

- **Elite athletes**
- **Children and adolescents**
- **Older adults**
- **Clinical patients**
- **Long-term users (5–10+ years)**

In all of these populations, creatine has shown:

- **No adverse effects on kidney or liver function** in healthy individuals
- **No increase in cardiovascular risk**
- **No link to dehydration, muscle cramps, or heat illness**
- **No negative effects on bone density or hormone levels**

A 2021 position paper from the **International Society of Sports Nutrition (ISSN)** concluded:

"Creatine monohydrate is the most effective ergogenic nutritional supplement currently available to athletes in terms of increasing high-intensity exercise capacity and lean body mass. Additionally, creatine has been shown to be safe across all populations when used appropriately."

This includes **daily use over years**, not just short-term cycles.

2. The Myth of Kidney Damage

Perhaps the most persistent myth about creatine is that it causes kidney damage. This myth stems from:

- **Confusion with creatinine**, a natural waste product measured in kidney function tests
- **Early case reports**, which lacked proper scientific controls

Let's clarify:

- Creatine is converted into **creatinine**, which is excreted via the kidneys.
- Supplementation may slightly raise **serum creatinine**, a marker used to estimate kidney function.

86

- **This does NOT indicate kidney damage.** It reflects increased creatine turnover, not reduced filtration.

In **dozens of clinical trials**, researchers have specifically monitored **blood urea nitrogen (BUN), glomerular filtration rate (GFR), and creatinine clearance**. None showed harmful effects on kidney function in healthy users.

However, individuals with **pre-existing kidney disease** should consult their healthcare provider before using creatine, as they may already have compromised filtration systems.

---

3. Bloating, Cramping, and Water Retention

Another common concern is that creatine causes:

- **Water retention**
- **Muscle cramping**
- **Bloating or stomach upset**

Let's examine the facts:

- Creatine causes **intracellular water retention** - meaning water is drawn into muscle cells, not under the skin. This is **beneficial**, as it supports performance and muscle volume.
- Modern dosing protocols (3–5 g/day) are **less likely to cause bloating** than older loading protocols (20 g/day).
- Muscle cramps are **not consistently reported** in scientific trials. In fact, several studies found **lower cramp rates** in creatine users during exercise or heat exposure.
- GI upset can occur, especially if taken in large doses or without enough water. This is **preventable** by splitting the dose and taking it with food or fluids.

In general, most side effects attributed to creatine are **mild, preventable, and rare** - especially with moderate dosing.

4. Creatine and Children or Adolescents

Creatine is one of the few performance-related supplements **studied in youth athletes and pediatric clinical populations**. Conditions studied include:

- **Muscular dystrophy**
- **Traumatic brain injury**
- **Sports performance in teens**

Findings consistently show:

- **No adverse effects** on growth, maturation, or organ health
- **Potential therapeutic benefits** in pediatric illness
- Enhanced **cognitive and physical performance** in teens under supervision

The **American Academy of Pediatrics** and ISSN agree that:

Creatine may be appropriate for adolescents involved in **serious training**, or for **clinical use**, under the guidance of qualified professionals.

Proper hydration, dosing, and education are essential, but **safety is well established** when used responsibly.

5. Interactions with Medications and Medical Conditions

Creatine is very well-tolerated, but users should be aware of potential **interactions or contraindications,** including:

Use caution or medical supervision if:

- You have **chronic kidney disease**
- You take **nephrotoxic medications** (e.g., some antibiotics, NSAIDs, diuretics)
- You have **severe liver disease**
- You are undergoing **dialysis or chemotherapy**

In these cases, creatine may still be usable but requires **routine monitoring** and medical approval.

Creatine is safe with:

- Blood pressure medications
- Antidepressants
- Statins and cholesterol drugs
- Thyroid medications
- Hormonal birth control
- Most over-the-counter pain relievers

Always disclose supplement use to your healthcare team - especially in surgery prep or disease management plans.

6. Is Creatine a Steroid? A Clarification

Another common myth is that creatine is a **steroid** or **hormone-like compound**. This is false.

Creatine is:

- A **naturally occurring compound** made from amino acids
- **Not a hormone**, nor does it affect testosterone or estrogen
- **Not classified as a controlled substance**
- Legal, widely available, and recognized as safe by sports and health organizations globally

Unlike anabolic steroids, creatine works by **enhancing cellular energy**, not by altering gene expression or hormonal pathways.

7. The Cleanest Form: Creatine Monohydrate

With the explosion of creatine products on the market, it's important to stick with the **safest and most studied form: creatine monohydrate**.

Avoid unproven variants like:

- Creatine ethyl ester (CEE)
- Liquid creatine
- Buffered creatine
- Creatine hydrochloride (HCl)

These versions are often:

- **More expensive**
- **Less effective**
- **Less studied**

Choose creatine monohydrate with **Creapure® certification** or other third-party testing for purity.

8. Long-Term Use and Cycling

Do you need to "cycle off" creatine?

No. There is no evidence that long-term daily use causes dependence, desensitization, or side effects.

- Continuous use of **3–5 grams/day** is safe and effective.
- You can stop at any time without withdrawal or rebound effects.
- Cycling is optional, but **not necessary** for safety.

Some users may choose to pause for budget or personal reasons, but there is **no physiological need** to take breaks if it continues to benefit you.

9. Environmental and Ethical Considerations

For those concerned with sustainability and animal welfare:

- Creatine supplements today are **synthetically produced** and **vegan-friendly**
- They do **not use animal tissue or byproducts**
- This makes creatine accessible to vegetarians, vegans, and ethically conscious users

It's also a **low-footprint supplement** - requiring minimal resources to manufacture, ship, and store.

10. Summary: One of the Safest Supplements Available

The safety of creatine is no longer up for debate. After decades of research, we now know:

- Creatine is **safe for healthy adults**, older adults, and clinical populations
- Myths about kidney damage, water retention, or hormonal disruption are **scientifically unfounded**
- When used properly, side effects are **rare, mild, and manageable**
- Long-term daily use is **well-supported** by evidence

Creatine isn't just safe - it's **reliably effective**, **clinically respected**, and **extraordinarily well-tolerated**.

Coming Up Next

In **Chapter 12: Dosing, Timing, and Stacking - How to Maximize Creatine's Benefits**, we'll get practical. You'll learn how to take creatine for specific goals (muscle, brain, metabolism), how to time it for maximum effect, and which nutrients or supplements pair best with it for full-body optimization.

Chapter 12: Dosing, Timing, and Stacking - How to Maximize Creatine's Benefits

Science-backed strategies for optimal results across every health and performance goal

Creatine has earned its reputation as a safe, effective, and versatile supplement. But to unlock its full potential, **how** you take it matters. The right dosage, timing, and combinations (also called "stacking") can significantly influence outcomes - whether your goal is enhanced cognition, muscle growth, mood stabilization, or disease support.

In this chapter, we'll outline a **goal-specific guide to creatine use** - detailing when to take it, how much to take, what to take it with, and how to combine it with other lifestyle factors or supplements for maximum synergy.

---

1. Creatine Forms: Stick With What Works

There are dozens of creatine formulations on the market, but research overwhelmingly supports **creatine monohydrate** as the gold standard. It's:

- The most **studied**
- The most **bioavailable**
- The most **cost-effective**
- The most **stable and shelf-safe**

You may encounter:

- Creatine HCl (hydrochloride)
- Creatine ethyl ester (CEE)
- Buffered creatines (e.g., Kre-Alkalyn)

- Liquid creatines

However, these alternatives:

- Are **less supported by evidence**
- Often **cost more without better results**
- May be **less stable or less absorbable**

Conclusion: Use **pure creatine monohydrate**, ideally from a **third-party-tested brand** (e.g., Creapure® certification).

---

2. General Dosing Guidelines

Maintenance Dose (Daily Use)

- **3 to 5 grams/day** for most adults
- Take **indefinitely** for continued benefit

Loading Phase (Optional)

- **20 grams/day**, split into 4 doses of 5g, for **5–7 days**
- Rapidly saturates muscle and brain stores
- Followed by **maintenance phase** of 3–5 grams/day

Higher Cognitive or Clinical Doses

- **5 to 10 grams/day**, especially during:
  - High stress
  - Sleep deprivation
  - Depression
  - Injury recovery
  - Brain training or rehabilitation

- Doses up to **20 g/day** have been used safely in short-term trials (e.g., for brain injury)

3. Best Time to Take Creatine

While timing is **not critical**, there are strategic advantages based on your goals:

For Physical Performance

- **Post-workout** with a meal or protein shake is best
    - Enhances muscle uptake via insulin response
    - May reduce soreness and support recovery

For Cognitive and Mood Benefits

- **Morning** or **before demanding mental tasks**
- Consistency is more important than time of day

For Sleep or Recovery Support

- **Evening dosing** may be helpful for those with fatigue, insomnia, or recovery needs

Pro tip: Creatine is not a stimulant. It will not keep you awake.

4. Should You Take It With Food?

Yes - especially with **carbohydrates or protein**.

Why?

- Insulin helps shuttle creatine into muscle and brain cells
- Meals improve gastrointestinal tolerance
- Stacking with carbs (e.g., fruit juice or a banana) enhances creatine retention

Avoid: Taking creatine on an empty stomach in large doses, which may cause bloating or cramping in sensitive individuals.

---

5. Creatine "Stacking": What Pairs Well?

Creatine works synergistically with several other supplements and nutrients. Some powerful combinations include:

Creatine + Protein

- Ideal for **muscle growth** and recovery
- Combine with **whey protein**, **plant protein**, or **collagen**

Creatine + Carbohydrates

- Enhances **muscle creatine uptake**
- Useful post-workout or for **glycogen replenishment**

Creatine + Omega-3s

- Supports **brain health and inflammation reduction**
- Combine for cognitive, mood, or neuroprotective benefits

Creatine + Magnesium

- Aids **muscle relaxation, ATP stability, and nervous system health**
- Especially helpful in **fatigue, sleep issues, or migraines**

Creatine + Alpha-Lipoic Acid (ALA)

- Improves **insulin sensitivity and creatine transport**
- May help with **Type 2 diabetes** and metabolic syndrome

Creatine + Vitamin D

- Supports **muscle and bone health**
- Vitamin D may also impact creatine kinase expression

6. Tailoring Creatine to Your Goal

For Muscle Growth & Performance

- 5g/day post-workout
- Combine with resistance training + protein + carbs

For Cognitive Support or Brain Health

- 5–10g/day
- Combine with omega-3s, B-vitamins, antioxidants

For Mood or Mental Health

- 5g/day with food
- Pair with SSRIs (if prescribed) or therapy protocols

For Older Adults (Fall Prevention, Frailty)

- 3–5g/day daily with meals
- Combine with low-impact strength training

For Chronic Illness or Recovery

- 5g/day minimum
- Work with a provider for higher or therapeutic dosing

7. Creatine Cycling: Do You Need It?

No.
Creatine does **not require cycling on or off**. The benefits persist with continued use, and there is:

- No evidence of dependence
- No tolerance buildup
- No suppression of natural creatine production

However, **you can cycle** if desired - for example:

- 8 weeks on, 4 weeks off
- 6 months on, 1 month off
- This may help reassess need or reduce supplement fatigue

8. Hydration and Creatine

Because creatine **pulls water into cells**, it's important to:

- Stay **well-hydrated**
- Drink **at least 2–3 liters** of water per day, especially if active
- Monitor for **muscle tightness** or **dehydration** during hot weather

This is not dangerous - but proper hydration optimizes performance and prevents rare side effects.

9. Is Timing Critical for Everyone?

Not always. For general users:

- **Consistency trumps timing**
- It's more important to **take creatine every day** than to worry about the exact hour

That said, pairing it with your **most physically or cognitively demanding task** may provide a noticeable edge in energy or stamina.

10. Creatine in Different Populations

Women

- May benefit from **lower doses** (3g/day), but respond well to higher ones during:
  - PMS
  - Pregnancy (pending medical approval)
  - Perimenopause or menopause
- Pair with resistance training for **muscle, bone, and mood benefits**

Vegans & Vegetarians

- Often respond **more dramatically** to supplementation
- Aim for 5g/day regularly
- Consider **loading phase** to saturate stores faster

Older Adults

- Creatine improves **frailty, balance, bone integrity, and cognition**
- Safe for long-term use (3–5g/day)

- Combine with **functional exercise**, such as walking, stairs, or light resistance

Summary: Make Creatine Work for You

Creatine is versatile, safe, and incredibly effective - but to unlock its full power:

- Use the **right dose** for your goals
- Pair it with the **right nutrients**
- Take it **consistently**
- Stack it with **exercise, sleep, and hydration**

Whether you're trying to lift more, think clearer, age stronger, or heal faster, creatine fits almost every health and performance strategy - and it adapts to your body, your diet, and your goals.

Coming Up Next

In **Chapter 13: Creatine and the Brain - Fuel for Focus, Memory, and Mood**, we'll zoom in on the central nervous system and explore how creatine protects and powers your brain, boosts your memory and mental clarity, and may play a key role in psychological resilience and neurodegenerative defense.

Chapter 13: The Longevity Molecule - Creatine and Healthy Aging

How one simple compound helps preserve vitality, cognition, and independence into later life

Aging is inevitable - but the **rate and quality** of aging are highly modifiable.

While many people associate aging with weakness, forgetfulness, and decline, the reality is that **biological aging can be slowed**. The key lies in preserving:

- Muscle mass and strength
- Cognitive clarity
- Bone integrity
- Cellular energy
- Resilience against disease

Remarkably, **creatine supports all of these dimensions**.

In this chapter, we explore how creatine becomes a powerful, science-backed tool for **healthy aging**, helping older adults not just survive - but thrive - with energy, strength, and independence.

1. The Challenge of Aging: A Loss of Reserves

Aging is characterized by:

- **Loss of lean muscle (sarcopenia)**
- **Decreased bone density**
- **Cognitive decline**
- **Increased inflammation and oxidative stress**

- **Mitochondrial dysfunction** (lower ATP production)

Together, these changes contribute to:

- **Falls, fractures, and frailty**
- **Fatigue and depression**
- **Reduced mobility and independence**
- **Higher risk for diseases like Alzheimer's, diabetes, and heart disease**

Many of these age-related declines can be **delayed or reversed** with the right interventions. Creatine stands out because it **supports the key systems that aging challenges most**.

2. Muscle Mass, Strength, and Function

Sarcopenia - age-related muscle loss - affects up to **50% of adults over 70** and is a major cause of:

- Weakness
- Loss of balance
- Impaired mobility
- Reduced metabolism
- Frailty-related hospitalizations

Creatine's benefits for muscle in aging adults:

- Increases **lean muscle mass**
- Enhances **muscle fiber size and strength**
- Improves **power output** (e.g., rising from a chair, climbing stairs)
- Supports **walking speed and gait stability**
- Reduces **fall risk**

When combined with **resistance training**, creatine **amplifies muscle gains** - especially in people over 60.

Meta-analyses show that older adults using creatine:

- Gain significantly more **strength and muscle** vs. placebo
- Improve **functional performance** (e.g., chair stand, timed walking)
- Maintain **mobility and independence** longer into old age

3. Bone Health and Fracture Prevention

Osteoporosis and osteopenia become common with age - especially in **postmenopausal women** and sedentary adults.

As covered in Chapter 8, creatine:

- Enhances **bone geometry and density** (especially in hips and femur)
- Supports **osteoblast activity** (cells that build bone)
- Improves **neuromuscular strength**, reducing fracture risk from falls

Studies show that **creatine + resistance exercise** helps preserve:

- **Hip and spine bone mineral density**
- **Functional movement and joint stability**
- **Postural strength** to prevent accidental falls

4. Cognition, Memory, and Mental Clarity

Cognitive aging is marked by:

- Slower processing speed
- Memory lapses
- Executive function decline
- Increased risk of **dementia and neurodegeneration**

Creatine plays a critical role in:

- Preserving **brain energy metabolism**
- Improving **working memory and attention**
- Enhancing **mental stamina** (especially under fatigue or stress)
- Supporting **neurotransmitter balance** and **neuronal protection**

Studies have found that:

- **Older adults supplementing with creatine** perform better on memory and logic tasks
- Creatine helps protect against **age-related brain volume shrinkage**
- Supplementation can reduce **brain fog** and **emotional instability**

When paired with **cognitive training** or a brain-healthy lifestyle (e.g., Mediterranean diet, social engagement), creatine magnifies brain resilience.

5. Cardiometabolic Health and Inflammation

With age comes an increased risk for:

- **High blood pressure**
- **Elevated blood glucose**
- **High triglycerides**
- **Systemic inflammation**

Creatine helps mitigate these risks by:

- **Improving endothelial function** (blood vessel health)
- Enhancing **glucose tolerance and insulin sensitivity**
- Lowering **triglyceride levels** in older adults
- Reducing **inflammatory markers** like CRP and TNF-α

These changes lead to:

- Improved **cardiovascular flexibility**
- Lower **metabolic disease risk**
- Better **vascular delivery of nutrients to muscles and the brain**

6. Psychological Well-being

Mental health is often overlooked in aging, yet depression, anxiety, and isolation are all too common in older populations.

Creatine may support psychological resilience by:

- Improving **mood and motivation**
- Enhancing **response to antidepressants**
- Reducing **fatigue and apathy**
- Supporting **emotional regulation** under stress

This is especially relevant for:

- **Postmenopausal women**
- **Older adults with mobility limitations**
- **Caregivers experiencing burnout**
- Individuals with **cognitive or physical comorbidities**

---

7. Immune Support and Recovery

As immune function declines with age, older adults become more vulnerable to:

- Infections (e.g., pneumonia, influenza)
- Slower wound healing
- Reduced recovery from surgery or injury

Creatine may:

- **Boost immune cell energy metabolism**
- Support **white blood cell function**
- Enhance **recovery from illness or hospitalization**
- Reduce **muscle catabolism** during bed rest or injury

In this way, creatine contributes to a **faster bounce-back** after health setbacks.

8. Creatine as a Longevity Supplement

Because of its **multi-system benefits**, creatine is being proposed as part of a **pro-longevity nutritional strategy**. It addresses several hallmarks of aging:

- **Mitochondrial dysfunction**
- **Cellular energy decline**
- **Inflammatory signaling**
- **Loss of proteostasis (muscle protein balance)**
- **Neurodegeneration**

No supplement is a "fountain of youth," but creatine comes close in its ability to:

- Maintain **strength and independence**
- Support **cognitive vitality**
- Protect against **falls and frailty**
- Improve **metabolic and immune resilience**

9. Safe, Simple, and Affordable

Perhaps the best part of creatine's longevity benefits is that it is:

- **Safe** for daily, long-term use in older adults
- **Easy to take** (3–5 grams/day with meals)
- **Affordable** compared to most anti-aging therapies
- Compatible with other interventions like:
  - **Strength training**
  - **Walking programs**
  - **Protein intake optimization**
  - **Vitamin D, B12, and omega-3s**

Creatine can be started at any age - but the earlier and more consistently it's used, the more benefits you accrue over time.

10. Ideal Aging Protocol with Creatine

Daily Creatine Plan for Adults 50+:

- **3–5 grams/day** (powder or capsule)
- Take with **a meal** or small carb source
- Combine with:
    - **Resistance or mobility training** (2–3x/week)
    - **Omega-3 fatty acids**
    - **Adequate protein (1.2–1.5g/kg/day)**
    - **Vitamin D3** (for muscle/bone synergy)

Consistency is key. Unlike fast-acting medications, creatine builds **quietly and powerfully over time**.

Summary: Age Strong, Think Sharp, Live Fully

Aging doesn't have to mean slowing down, giving up, or fading away. With the right choices, you can build a future filled with:

- **Strength**
- **Vitality**
- **Clarity**
- **Confidence**
- **Independence**

Creatine is one of the most powerful tools in that toolkit - supporting your muscles, brain, bones, heart, and mood as you age.

No gimmicks. No magic. Just science, consistency, and a molecule your body already understands.

Coming Up Next

In **Chapter 14: Your Creatine Blueprint - A Lifestyle Guide for Long-Term Vitality**, we'll tie everything together with clear action plans, checklists, and personalized strategies for integrating creatine into your life - no matter your age, gender, diet, or goals.

Chapter 14: Your Creatine Blueprint - A Lifestyle Guide for Long-Term Vitality

Personalized plans, daily practices, and holistic strategies for maximizing creatine's impact

By now, you've learned that **creatine is more than just a supplement for athletes** - it's a cellular powerhouse that supports nearly every system in your body: muscles, brain, bones, metabolism, and mood.

But information alone doesn't create transformation. The final chapter of this book is your **action guide** - a personalized, practical blueprint for integrating creatine into your life in a way that supports **energy, strength, clarity, and health - every day, for the long haul**.

Whether you're 25 or 75, sedentary or active, healthy or healing, the strategies here will help you **activate creatine's full potential** in your body and mind.

1. Start with "Why": Define Your Primary Goal

Creatine supports many outcomes, but your implementation should start with a **clear purpose**. Ask yourself:

"What do I want creatine to do for me?"

Some common goals include:

- Build or maintain muscle
- Improve memory, focus, or mental clarity
- Support mood, motivation, or emotional resilience
- Age with strength, independence, and vitality
- Improve heart, metabolic, or joint health
- Boost performance in sports or training

- Recover from illness, fatigue, or injury

Write this goal down. It will help you stick with your plan and track your progress.

2. Choose Your Creatine Type

Use Creatine Monohydrate - always.

- Scientifically validated
- Affordable
- Stable and pure
- Suitable for long-term use
- Vegan and synthetic (not derived from animals)

Look for:

- **Creapure®** or other third-party tested certifications
- Powder or capsule form (whichever you'll take consistently)
- Avoid gimmicks like "liquid creatine" or "special blends" - they're more expensive, not more effective

3. Personalize Your Daily Dose

Your Goal	Daily Dose
General health / muscle support	3–5g/day
Brain + mood + stress resilience	5–10g/day
Aging support / anti-frailty	5g/day
High-intensity athletics	5–10g/day
Recovery from illness or injury	5g/day
Vegans/vegetarians	5g/day

Optional loading phase: 20g/day (split in 4 doses) for 5–7 days, then return to maintenance dose.

Take with:

- A **meal**, preferably with **carbs or protein**
- Plenty of water (especially during the loading phase)

4. Timing Strategies Based on Lifestyle

If you train regularly:

- Take **post-workout** with a protein shake or carb-rich snack

If cognitive clarity is your goal:

- Take **first thing in the morning**, optionally again in the early afternoon

If you struggle with sleep or fatigue:

- Try **evening dosing** to reduce energy dips during recovery

If you're over 50:

- Take creatine **with breakfast or lunch** to help digestion and absorption

Consistency matters **more than time of day**, so focus on daily use above all.

5. Stack Creatine with Lifestyle and Nutrition

Creatine works best when combined with **supportive habits**. Build your daily "stack" with:

Movement

- Resistance training 2–4x/week
- Walking, stretching, or yoga on rest days
- Balance and mobility work if over 50

Nutrition

- Protein-rich meals (1.2–1.6g/kg/day)
- Omega-3 fats (fish, chia, walnuts, or supplements)
- Colorful veggies and berries (for antioxidant support)
- Hydration: at least **2–3 liters of water/day**

Mind-Body Balance

- Sleep: 7–9 hours
- Stress reduction: breathwork, meditation, nature, journaling
- Social connection: friendships and purpose fuel health, too

Optional Supplement Pairings

- **Vitamin D3 + K2** (bone and mood synergy)
- **Magnesium** (muscle, mood, and ATP support)
- **B-complex vitamins** (especially for vegetarians and over-60s)
- **Omega-3s** (brain and inflammation support)

6. Monitoring Your Progress

Creatine's effects are subtle at first - but **accumulative and powerful** over time.

Track changes like:

- Strength improvements
- Mental clarity and productivity
- Mood stability and energy levels
- Recovery after exercise or stressful days
- Mobility, balance, and physical confidence
- Sleep quality and emotional resilience

Consider taking **baseline notes**, then check in weekly or monthly.

Creatine doesn't "kick in" like a stimulant - it builds your body's **resilience from the inside out**.

7. Special Considerations by Population

Older Adults:

- May benefit from **higher doses (5g daily)** for sarcopenia, cognition, and energy
- Combine with resistance bands, walking, or tai chi
- Monitor fall risk, mobility, and fatigue improvements

Vegans and Vegetarians:

- Have **lower baseline creatine stores**
- Often experience **more dramatic improvements**
- 5g/day is ideal (optional loading recommended)

Women:

- Safe across the lifespan
- May reduce PMS symptoms and emotional fluctuations
- Useful during **perimenopause and menopause** for muscle, mood, and cognition

People with Chronic Conditions:

- Work with a healthcare provider for tailored dosing
- Creatine may help with fatigue, pain, inflammation, and healing
- Especially helpful for people with **fibromyalgia**, **mood disorders**, or **neuromuscular issues**

8. Addressing Common Questions

Q: Can I take creatine forever?
Yes - long-term use is **safe, effective, and supported by research**.

Q: Should I stop during vacation or travel?
Not unless you want to. Creatine is safe and simple to travel with.

Q: Can I use it if I don't exercise?
Absolutely. Even without training, creatine supports **brain, bone, and metabolic health**.

Q: Is it safe with medications?
Generally yes, but always consult your doctor - especially if you have **kidney issues or take diuretics**.

Q: What if I miss a day?
No problem. Just resume the next day. It's about **long-term consistency**, not perfection.

9. Final Thoughts: Your Body's Best Ally

If there were a supplement that could:

- Build strength
- Enhance cognition
- Protect your brain
- Improve your mood
- Lower your risk for chronic disease
- And support graceful aging...

...and it cost pennies a day, was safe for nearly everyone, and was already present in your body - **wouldn't you want it?**

That's creatine.

Simple. Proven. Powerful. And now, yours to use with purpose and confidence.

Your Action Checklist

Define your goal
Choose high-quality creatine monohydrate
Start with 3–5g/day (up to 10g/day for cognitive or clinical goals)
Take consistently with meals
Combine with resistance training and brain-nourishing habits
Stack with hydration, sleep, and supportive nutrients
Track your progress and make it your own

Closing Words

This book was designed to not only **educate you**, but to **empower you** - to take ownership of your health with one of the most accessible and effective tools in modern wellness.

Creatine is not a trend. It's a **timeless molecule**, essential for life and renewal, now supported by cutting-edge science and real-world results.

Wherever you are in your journey - rebuilding, leveling up, aging with intention - **creatine belongs in your story**.

You are not fragile. You are energy. You are strength. You are made to move, think, and thrive.

Let creatine help you do exactly that.

Chapter 15: Final Thoughts — Creatine as a Pillar of 21st Century Health

Where We've Been — and Where Creatine Can Take Us

As we bring this book to a close, it's worth pausing to recognize how far our understanding of creatine has come—and how much it still has to offer.

Once dismissed as "just a gym supplement," creatine is now recognized for what it truly is: **a foundational molecule for human energy, function, and resilience**. It is supported by hundreds of peer-reviewed studies, celebrated for its broad safety profile, and backed by an evolving body of clinical research that spans physical, cognitive, and emotional health.

In this final chapter, we'll synthesize what you've learned and help you turn information into action. Whether you're looking to boost brainpower, support healthy aging, maintain muscle mass, or simply feel more energized day to day, creatine can—and should—be part of your long-term wellness strategy.

Creatine at a Glance: One Molecule, Many Benefits

Let's quickly revisit the multi-system power of creatine supplementation:

System	Benefits of Creatine
Muscles & Bones	Increases strength and power, supports muscle retention, improves recovery, and may enhance bone density.
Brain & Mood	Supports mental clarity, memory, focus, and may reduce symptoms of depression, anxiety, and cognitive fatigue.
Aging	Counters muscle and brain decline, reduces frailty risk, supports independence and quality of life.
Metabolism & Heart	May improve glucose tolerance, cardiovascular output, and support mitochondrial health.
Hormonal Health	Helps women during PMS, pregnancy, postpartum, and menopause by supporting mood, cognition, and energy levels.

Summary by Age & Lifestyle Group

Children / Teens (Under Clinical Supervision Only)

Creatine can benefit youth in athletic development, especially in sports, or in rare clinical cases of creatine deficiency syndromes. Always consult a pediatric physician first.

Young Adults & Students (18–30)

Why it matters: High mental stress, poor sleep, and cognitive overload are common.

Benefits: Improved memory, sharper focus, less mental fatigue, better athletic performance.

Use: 3–5 g/day of creatine monohydrate, with or without a loading phase.

Professionals / Busy Adults (30–50)

Why it matters: Career, parenting, and burnout can drain energy and focus.

Benefits: Mood support, enhanced cognition, energy recovery, muscle preservation.

Use: Daily dosing; consider pairing with brain-healthy habits (hydration, sleep, mindfulness).

Adults Over 50 / Retirees

Why it matters: Age-related loss of muscle and brain function accelerates.

Benefits: Slower physical decline, cognitive protection, greater mobility and independence.

Use: Start with 3–5 g/day; combine with light resistance training for maximum benefit.

Vegetarians / Vegans

Why it matters: Creatine is absent in plant-based diets.

Benefits: Cognitive enhancement, muscle and energy support, stronger training outcomes.

Use: Especially responsive to supplementation; daily dosing highly recommended.

Women (All Life Stages)

Why it matters: Hormonal fluctuations impact energy, mood, and cognition.

Benefits: Eases PMS-related fatigue and mood swings, supports cognition in menopause and pregnancy.

Use: Daily dosing is safe and beneficial; especially valuable during hormonal transitions.

A Simple Checklist: Your Creatine Integration Plan

1. Choose the Right Type

- **Creatine Monohydrate** is the gold standard—proven, safe, and affordable.

2. Choose a Dosage

- Standard dose: **3–5 grams per day**
- Optional loading: **20 grams/day for 5–7 days**, then maintain at 3–5 grams

3. Choose a Time

- No need to obsess over timing.
- However, post-workout or with a carb-containing meal may improve absorption.

4. Stay Hydrated

- Creatine draws water into cells.
- Drink 6–8 glasses of water daily for optimal results and comfort.

5. Track Your Benefits

Keep a log of:

- Cognitive clarity
- Physical strength
- Mood and motivation
- Recovery time and sleep quality

Results may take **2–4 weeks** to become noticeable—stay consistent.

A Final Word on Safety

Creatine is one of the **most rigorously studied** dietary supplements in existence. According to the **International Society of Sports Nutrition**, long-term creatine use—even at high doses—has not been shown to cause kidney, liver, or muscle damage in healthy individuals.

Common myths debunked:

- Creatine does **not** cause kidney damage
- Creatine does **not** cause water retention in organs
- Creatine does **not** cause hair loss (evidence is anecdotal, not clinical)
- Creatine does **not** need to be cycled off

That said, anyone with **pre-existing kidney disease or metabolic disorders** should consult their doctor before use.

Creatine is Accessible, Affordable, and Adaptable

One of the best things about creatine? It's:

- **Inexpensive** (about $0.10–0.20 per day)
- **Widely available worldwide**
- **Vegan-friendly (synthetically produced creatine)**
- **Shelf-stable and mixable in nearly any beverage**

No prescription required. No complicated protocol. Just a powerful, simple addition to your daily wellness toolkit.

Creatine as a Pillar of 21st Century Health

In the 20th century, we emphasized disease treatment.
In the 21st century, we must prioritize **energy, prevention, and resilience**.

Creatine meets the moment:

- It supports **longevity** by protecting what declines most with age—muscle and brain.
- It enhances **everyday performance**, from mental focus to physical endurance.
- It's safe, studied, and sustainable.

In a world full of overhyped supplements, creatine stands apart: **a molecule your body already knows—but one that needs your support**.

Final Takeaway

If you're looking to:

- Feel sharper
- Move better
- Age stronger
- Stay emotionally balanced
- Protect your body and brain for the long haul...

Creatine might be the missing link.

It's time to stop thinking of creatine as a supplement.
It's time to start thinking of it as a pillar of modern health.

Bibliography

1. **Buford, T. W., Kreider, R. B., Stout, J. R., Greenwood, M., Campbell, B., Spano, M., ... & Antonio, J.** (2007). *International Society of Sports Nutrition position stand: creatine supplementation and exercise.* Journal of the International Society of Sports Nutrition, 4(1), 6.
https://doi.org/10.1186/1550-2783-4-6

2. **Kreider, R. B., Kalman, D. S., Antonio, J., Ziegenfuss, T. N., Wildman, R., Collins, R., & Lopez, H. L.** (2017). *International Society of Sports Nutrition position stand: safety and efficacy of creatine supplementation in exercise, sport, and medicine.* Journal of the International Society of Sports Nutrition, 14(1), 18.
https://doi.org/10.1186/s12970-017-0173-z

3. **Candow, D. G., & Chilibeck, P. D.** (2008). *Timing of creatine or protein supplementation and resistance training in the elderly.* Applied Physiology, Nutrition, and Metabolism, 33(1), 184-190.
https://doi.org/10.1139/H07-134

4. **Devries, M. C., Phillips, S. M.** (2014). *Creatine supplementation during resistance training in older adults - a meta-analysis.* Medicine and Science in Sports and Exercise, 46(6), 1194-1203.
https://doi.org/10.1249/MSS.0000000000000220

5. **Forbes, S. C., Candow, D. G., Ostojic, S. M., & Roberts, M. D.** (2022). *Creatine supplementation and aging: focus on sarcopenia, falls and functional performance.* Amino Acids, 54(4), 453–462.
https://doi.org/10.1007/s00726-021-03053-w

6. **Rae, C., Digney, A. L., McEwan, S. R., & Bates, T. C.** (2003). *Oral creatine monohydrate supplementation improves brain performance: a double–blind, placebo–controlled, cross–over trial.* Psychopharmacology, 167(3), 282–289.
https://doi.org/10.1007/s00213-003-1400-6

7. **Lyoo, I. K., Yoon, S., Kim, T. S., Hwang, J., Kim, J. E., Won, W., ... & Renshaw, P. F.** (2012). *A randomized, double-blind placebo-controlled trial of oral creatine monohydrate augmentation for enhanced response to a selective serotonin reuptake inhibitor in women with major depressive disorder.* The American Journal of Psychiatry, 169(9), 937–945. https://doi.org/10.1176/appi.ajp.2012.11081392

8. **Bender, A., & Klopstock, T.** (2016). *Creatine for neuroprotection in neurodegenerative disease: end of story?* Amino Acids, 48, 1929–1940. https://doi.org/10.1007/s00726-016-2266-0

9. **Rawson, E. S., & Venezia, A. C.** (2011). *Use of creatine in the elderly and evidence for effects on cognitive function in young and old.* Amino Acids, 40(5), 1349–1362. https://doi.org/10.1007/s00726-011-0855-9

10. **Lobo, D. M., Tritto, A. C. C., da Silva, L. R., de Oliveira, P. B., Benatti, F. B., Roschel, H., ... & Gualano, B.** (2015). *Effects of creatine supplementation on cognitive function of healthy individuals: A systematic review of randomized controlled trials.* Clinical Nutrition, 34(3), 505–513. https://doi.org/10.1016/j.clnu.2014.05.007

11. **Gualano, B., Rawson, E. S., Candow, D. G., & Chilibeck, P. D.** (2016). *Creatine supplementation in the aging population: effects on skeletal muscle, bone and brain.* Amino Acids, 48(8), 1793–1805. https://doi.org/10.1007/s00726-016-2180-9

12. **Robinson, T. M., Sewell, D. A., Hultman, E., & Greenhaff, P. L.** (2000). *Role of creatine and phosphocreatine in neuronal development and function.* Developmental Neuroscience, 22(5-6), 307–313. https://doi.org/10.1159/000017470

13. **Smith, R. N., Agharkar, A. S., & Gonzales, E. B.** (2014). *A review of creatine supplementation in age-related diseases: more than a supplement for athletes.* F1000Research, 3, 222. https://doi.org/10.12688/f1000research.5218.1

14. **van der Zee, E. A., et al.** (2021). *Creatine monohydrate: A clinically promising adjunct to neurorehabilitation.* Neuroscience & Biobehavioral Reviews, 127, 709–728. https://doi.org/10.1016/j.neubiorev.2021.05.002

15. **Persky, A. M., & Brazeau, G. A.** (2001). *Clinical pharmacology of the dietary supplement creatine monohydrate.* Pharmacological Reviews, 53(2), 161–176. https://pharmrev.aspetjournals.org/content/53/2/161

16. **Gualano, B., et al.** (2012). *Creatine supplementation: evaluating the potential role in diseases.* Current Neuropharmacology, 10(3), 271–279. https://doi.org/10.2174/157015912803217311

17. **Antonio, J., et al.** (2021). *Common questions and misconceptions about creatine supplementation: what does the scientific evidence really show?* Journal of the International Society of Sports Nutrition, 18(1), 13. https://doi.org/10.1186/s12970-021-00412-w

Glossary

Adenosine Triphosphate (ATP)

The primary energy molecule used by cells in the body. ATP fuels most cellular activities, including muscle contractions, brain function, and metabolism. Creatine helps regenerate ATP quickly during energy-demanding tasks.

Bioavailability

A measure of how effectively a nutrient or supplement is absorbed and used by the body. Creatine monohydrate has high bioavailability.

Bone Mineral Density (BMD)

A measure of the amount of minerals (primarily calcium) in a specific volume of bone. It is used to assess bone strength and the risk of fractures. Creatine may support BMD, especially in combination with resistance training.

Buffering Agent

A compound that helps stabilize pH in the body. Creatine can act as a buffering agent, helping to reduce the buildup of acid in muscles during high-intensity exercise.

Cognition

The set of mental processes related to knowledge, including attention, memory, language, problem-solving, and decision-making. Creatine has been shown to enhance various aspects of cognition, especially under stress.

Creatine

A naturally occurring compound made from amino acids, stored primarily in muscle cells and the brain. It helps rapidly regenerate ATP. Supplemental creatine is used to enhance strength, cognition, recovery, and overall health.

Creatine Monohydrate

The most studied and commonly used form of creatine. It is highly effective, safe, and affordable. Most clinical research supporting creatine's benefits uses this form.

Creatinine

A waste product formed by the breakdown of creatine in the body. Elevated creatinine levels in the blood can indicate kidney function, but increases due to creatine supplementation do not necessarily mean kidney damage.

Ergogenic Aid

A substance that enhances physical performance. Creatine is considered one of the most effective ergogenic aids for improving strength, power, and endurance.

Executive Function

Cognitive processes that manage and regulate other abilities and behaviors, such as planning, focusing attention, remembering instructions, and juggling multiple tasks.

Glomerular Filtration Rate (GFR)

A test used to check how well the kidneys are filtering blood. Often referenced in creatine studies to monitor kidney health.

Intracellular Water Retention

Water that is drawn into the inside of cells (such as muscle cells), which is a normal effect of creatine. It is not the same as bloating or subcutaneous water retention.

Loading Phase

A short-term strategy for saturating the body's creatine stores quickly. Typically involves taking 20 grams/day (divided into 4 doses) for 5–7 days before switching to a maintenance dose.

Maintenance Dose

The regular, ongoing dose of creatine (usually 3–5 grams/day) taken after a loading phase or used as a long-term routine.

Mitochondria

Organelles within cells that produce energy (ATP). Sometimes referred to as the "powerhouses" of the cell. Creatine supports mitochondrial efficiency and function.

Mood Regulation

The process by which the brain manages emotional states. Creatine contributes to mood stability by supporting energy availability and neurotransmitter production.

Neurodegeneration

The progressive loss of structure or function of neurons, leading to conditions such as Alzheimer's, Parkinson's, and ALS. Creatine may offer neuroprotective benefits.

Neuroprotection

Interventions or substances that help preserve the function and structure of neurons. Creatine is studied for its neuroprotective effects in aging and disease.

Nootropic

A substance that enhances cognitive performance, especially executive functions, memory, and focus. Creatine is considered a natural nootropic in certain contexts.

Oxidative Stress

Damage to cells caused by reactive oxygen species (free radicals). This process contributes to aging and various diseases. Creatine helps reduce oxidative stress through mitochondrial support.

Phosphocreatine System

A cellular energy system in which stored creatine phosphate donates a phosphate group to ADP to rapidly regenerate ATP during short bursts of high energy demand.

Placebo-Controlled Trial

A scientific study in which one group receives the treatment (e.g., creatine), and another group receives a placebo. It helps determine the true effect of the supplement.

Resistance Training

Exercise that causes muscles to contract against an external resistance (e.g., weights or bands), improving strength and muscle mass. Creatine works synergistically with resistance training.

Sarcopenia

The age-related loss of muscle mass, strength, and function. Creatine has been shown to help prevent or slow the progression of sarcopenia.

Sleep Deprivation

A state caused by insufficient sleep. It impairs cognitive and physical performance. Creatine can help mitigate the negative effects of sleep loss on the brain.

Stacking

The practice of combining creatine with other supplements or nutrients (like protein or omega-3s) to enhance results.

Supplementation

The act of taking additional nutrients (like creatine) in addition to a regular diet, usually to support health, performance, or specific goals.

Vegan / Vegetarian Diets

Diets that avoid (or minimize) animal products. Individuals on these diets typically have lower creatine stores due to reduced dietary intake, and may benefit significantly from supplementation.